I. Rocker (Ed.)

Pelvic Pain in Women
Diagnosis and Management

Foreword by L.P. Thomas

With 32 Figures

Springer-Verlag
London Berlin Heidelberg New York
Paris Tokyo Hong Kong

I. Rocker, MD, FRCOG
Consultant Obstetrician and Gynaecologist, Royal Gwent
Hospital, Newport, Gwent, NP9 2UB

British Library Cataloguing in Publication Data
Pelvic pain in women: diagnosis and management
    1. Women. Pelvis. Pain. diagnosis & relief
    I. Rocker, I.
    616.7'1

Library of Congress Cataloging-in-Publication Data
Pelvic pain in women: diagnosis and management. I. Rocker (ed.); foreword by
L.P. Thomas
    p. cm

    1. Pelvic pain. 2. Generative organs. Female—Diseases.
I. Rocker, I.
    [DNLM: 1. Genital Diseases, Female—diagnosis. 2. Genital Diseases,
    Female—therapy. 3. Pain—diagnosis. 4. Pain—therapy. 5. Pelvis.
    WP 140 D5359]
    RG483.P44D53   1989
    618. 1—dc20
    DNLM/DLC
    for Library of Congress   89–26181
                                                                  CIP

ISBN-13: 978-1-4471-3292-9   e-ISBN-13: 978-1-4471-3290-5
DOI: 10.1007/ 978-1-4471-3290-5

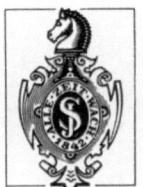

Foreword

Pelvic pain in the female patient is common in gynaecological practice, but the specialties of general surgery, urology and orthopaedics provide a significant number of patients and problems. These patients may suffer a multitude of symptoms, and only careful analysis and investigation of each individual problem by the doctor concerned will lead to correct diagnosis and management.

The subject matter of this book lies in the practice of many specialties, and all are combined here in a coherent whole. This emphasises the close collaboration necessary between family practitioners, junior hospital staff and consultants. The authors are consultants who work together in a busy district general hospital, and their experience and collaboration is evident in the approach to the diagnosis and management of pelvic pain in the female. Emphasis is laid on the careful evaluation of history and examination and the correct interpretation of diagnostic investigations. Full details of radiology, ultrasound scanning, endoscopy, peritoneoscopy and bacteriological investigation are given. Full consultation between members of staff who have special experience in these investigative procedures is of paramount importance. Details of treatment for relief of pain are important to all doctors concerned with this aspect of clinical management, and this section will be of particular value. The blending of these specialties allows full consideration of the problems affecting the patients. Careful management leads to better treatment for the patient and better satisfaction for the doctor.

Acute pelvic pain is easier to diagnose than chronic pain, and management is often more straightforward. Careful attention has been paid to the consideration of chronic pain with a multitude of symptoms. The psychological aspect of these problems is also fully covered, with emphasis on the consideration of the whole woman and her worries. The authors show considerable understanding of the difficult and sometimes delicate problems involved.

The book is directed to family practitioners, junior hospital doctors and medical students, and it is hoped that the full consideration of the many facets of pelvic pain will lead to a better understanding of the condition.

Newport, 1989   L. P. Thomas, M Ch, FRCS

Preface

Female pelvic pain is a common medical problem which in its acute, recurrent or chronic effects taxes the diagnostic and communication skills of all associated with patient care.

The changing pattern of life over the past 30 years has reduced parity and subsequent prolapse. Antibiotic therapy has changed the natural history of pelvic inflammatory disease, so that the inoperable frozen pelvis of the 1950s is now rarely encountered. Effective contraception has played a part in the increasing incidence of sexually transmitted disease and cervical intraepithelial neoplasia. While the number of live born has fallen in the past 20 years, there has been an increase in elective terminations of pregnancy, which now number 1 in 4 or 1 in 5 of all pregnancies. In addition there has been a rise in the number of one-parent families and their attendant social problems. Endometriosis is increasing in prevalence, and ovarian malignancy and bowel cancer have become, respectively, the commonest gynaecological and second commonest intestinal causes of death. There is also the additional expectation of diagnosis leading to treatment.

The primary health team successfully manages the majority of these problems, possibly with the backup of specialist services, but there remains a residual group of women who have chronic pelvic pain without obvious cause or acceptable explanation.

This handbook is the result of the combined experience of hospital consultants working in a large district general hospital, an association that for some began in their medical student days and for others 15 to 25 years ago. They have therefore coordinated their approach not only by cross referral but also by their teaching to graduate and postgraduate students. This book is intended as a guide for the management of common problems and particularly as a basis for communication to reduce the risk of vague explanation given in good faith but which increases anxiety.

My thanks are due to my colleagues for their willing cooperation, to Mrs Val Reed for the typing and to the Medical Illustration Department of the Royal Gwent Hospital for their sterling efforts.

Newport, 1989   I. Rocker

Contents

1 **General Aspects** 1

General Anatomy and Innervation of the Female Pelvis
D.E. Sturdy 1
   Innervation of the Pelvic Viscera.......................... 3
   Surgical Aspects of Female Pelvic Pain................. 5
   Gynaecological/Obstetric Aspects of Pelvic Pain....... 6

Neurophysiology of Pain
G.D. Thomas 6
   Neuroanatomy and Physiology 6
   Neuropeptides 9
   Application of Neurophysiology and Anatomy......... 10

Psychological Aspects of Pelvic Pain
J.M. Hughes 13
   Psychosomatic Medicine 13
   The Psychology of Pain 14
   Pelvic Pain in Women.. 14
   The Approach to Cancer and Cancerophobia.......... 17
   Standard Drugs Used in Psychiatry........................ 18

2 **Examination and Investigation** 21

General and Surgical Examination
D.E. Sturdy 21
   Examination for Acute Painful Conditions of the
      Perineum 21
   Examination for Acute Pelvic Pain........................ 22
   Examination for Chronic Pelvic Pain..................... 23

Gynaecological Examination and Investigation
I. Rocker 26

Gynaecological History 26
Gynaecological Examination 28

Orthopaedic Examination
D.G. Jones 30

Bacteriological Investigation of Genitourinary Infections
E.J.G. Glencross 31
    Urinary Tract Infection 31
    Vaginal Discharge 34
    Important Sexually Transmitted Diseases 35
    Pelvic Inflammatory Disease 38
    Chronic Pelvic Infection 40
    Summary of Common Diagnostic
        Specimens 40

Diagnostic Imaging
A. Jones 40
    Gynaecological Disease 41
    Urinary Tract Disease 45
    Intestinal Disease 49
    Skeletal Disease 54
    Computed Tomography in Pelvic Disease 55
    Radiological Intervention Techniques 56

Laparoscopy
I. Rocker 56
    Hysteroscopy 58

3   Reproduction and Pain
    I. Rocker 59
    Preadolescence 59
    Trauma 61
    Congenital Malformations 62
        Cysts and Tumours 62
    Dysmenorrhoea 63
    Sexual Activity and Pelvic Pain 68
        Dyspareunia 68
    Pregnancy 69
        Uterine Contractility and Labour 71
        The Ovary in Pregnancy 72
        Abnormalities of Intrauterine Pregnancy 73
        Trophoblastic Disease 74
        Ectopic Gestation 75
        Placental Abruption 76
        Gynaecological Problems and Pregnancy 77

4 Vulva, Vagina and Perineum 81

Vulva and Vagina
I. Rocker 81
   Trauma 81
   Infections 82
   Vulval Tumours 84
   Vulval Dystrophy/Dermatoses 84
   Vaginal Tumours 85
   Vaginal Cervix 85

Perineum
D.E. Sturdy 86
   Acute Painful Conditions of the Perineum 86
   Chronic Painful Conditions of the Perineum 89

5 Bladder and Renal Tract
D.E. Sturdy 93
Pain in the Anterior (Urinary) Compartment of the
   Female Pelvis 93
   Urethral Caruncle 93
   Acute Bladder Pain 94
   Chronic Bladder Pain 94
   Pain in the Intrapelvic Ureter 99
   Acute Ureteric Pain 99
   Chronic Ureteric Pain 101

6 Gynaecological Pain
I. Rocker 103
Uterovaginal Prolapse 103
Uterine Malposition 105
Pelvic Inflammatory Disease 109
Endometriosis 112
Genital Tract Tumours and Pelvic and Abdomino-
   pelvic Swellings 117
Uterine Enlargement 120
Post-hysterectomy Pain 123
Gynaecalgia 127

7 Surgical and Orthopaedic Causes of Pelvic Pain 133

Surgical Causes of Pelvic Pain
D.E. Sturdy 133
   Acute Intestinal Inflammation 133
   Pelvic Abscess 134
   Acute Intestinal Ischaemia and Obstruction 135
   Herniae 136

Chronic Inflammatory Bowel Disease 136
Stoma Management 142
Spasmodic Intestinal Disorders Producing Pelvic
  Pain 143
Neoplasms of the Large Bowel 143
Vascular Disorders Producing Pelvic Pain 148

Orthopaedic Causes of Pelvic Pain
D.G. Jones 150
Posterior Pelvic Pain 151
Anterior Pelvic Problems 152
Generalised Diseases Affecting the Pelvis 155

8 Pain Management
G.D. Thomas 157
Mild Pain 157
Moderate Pain 158
Severe Pain 158
Acute Pain 158
Chronic Pain 160

Further Reading 163

Subject Index 165

Contributors

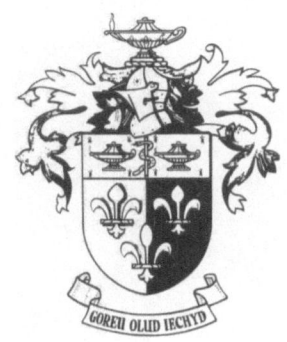

E.J.G. Glencross, MB, FRCPath
Consultant Bacteriologist

J.M. Hughes, BSc, FRCP, FRCPsych
Consultant Psychiatrist

A. Jones, MB, FRCR
Consultant Radiologist

D.G. Jones, MB, MRCP, FRCS
Consultant Orthopaedic Surgeon

I. Rocker, MD, FRCOG
Consultant Obstetrician and Gynaecologist

D.E. Sturdy, MS, FRCS
Consultant Surgeon and Urologist

G.D. Thomas, MB, FCAnaes
Consultant Anaesthetist

All contributors practise at the Royal Gwent Hospital, Newport,
Gwent, NP9 2UB.

1 General Aspects

J.M. HUGHES, D.E. STURDY and G.D. THOMAS

General Anatomy and Innervation of the Female Pelvis

D. E. Sturdy

The female pelvis is a basin-shaped cavity bounded anteriorly by the pubic bone, laterally by the ilium and ischium and posteriorly by the sacrum and coccyx (the true or lesser pelvis). The pelvic cavity is in direct communication with the abdominal cavity, and its upper limits are the tips of the iliac crests (the transtrochanteric line) related anteriorly to a surface point 3 to 4 cm below the umbilicus and posteriorly to the upper border of the fifth lumbar vertebra (Fig. 1.1). Its anterior wall is part of the musculature of the abdominal cavity. The lateral walls of the pelvic cavity are covered by the iliopsoas, iliacus and obturator muscles, and inferiorly the outlet is guarded by the levator ani and pubococcygeus muscles, which, with the corresponding muscles of the opposite side, form the pelvic diaphragm. Passing through this muscular diaphragm are three channels which open into the perineum, i.e. the urethra anteriorly, the vagina in the middle and the anal canal posteriorly. Anatomically, the visceral contents of the female pelvis can be separated into three compartments – anterior (urinary), middle (genital) and posterior (intestinal).

Within the pelvic basin the bladder and urethra lie anteriorly; the vagina, uterus, broad ligaments, Fallopian tubes and ovaries in the middle; and the anal canal and rectum posteriorly (Fig. 1.2). In addition, within its cavity, the pelvis contains loops of ileum, the sigmoid colon and frequently the greater omentum, the caecum and vermiform appendix. The ureter is the only structure which traverses from one compartment to the other. In its course along the lateral wall of the pelvis it lies in the middle compartment in close proximity to the ovary and in its terminal 4 cm it sweeps anteriorly into the anterior compartment. In this part of its course it is closely related to the lateral fornix of the vagina, especially on the left side. The interior

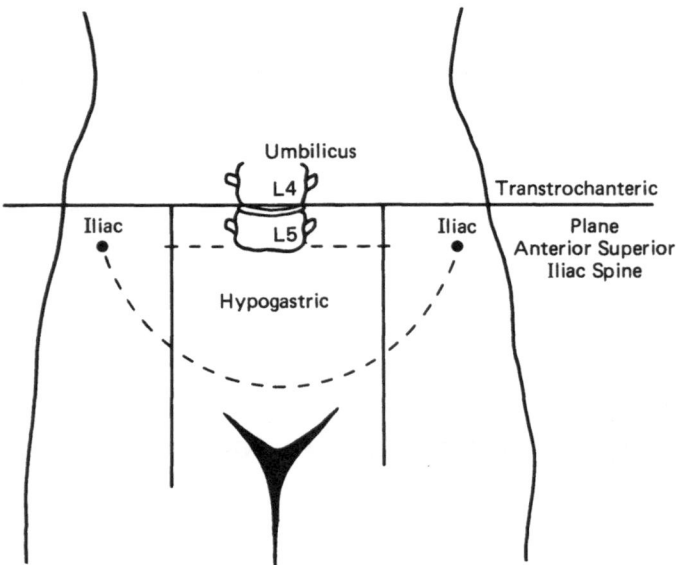

Fig. 1.1. Surface projection of upper limits of pelvis.

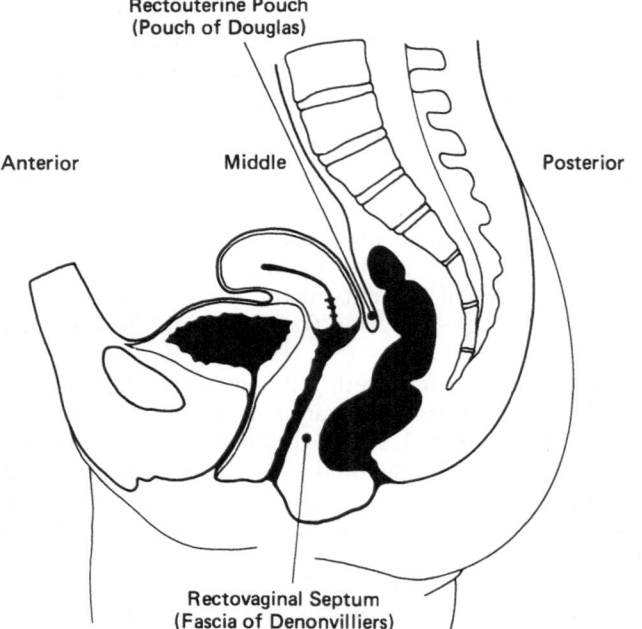

Fig. 1.2. Vertical section of female pelvis; compartmentalisation of pelvic viscera.

of the pelvic cavity is lined with peritoneum, which sweeps downwards on the internal surface of the anterior abdominal wall to cover the upper third of the bladder, the main bulk of the body of the uterus (forming the broad ligament which ensheathes the Fallopian tubes) and the anterior surface of the upper third of the rectum. At the rectosigmoid junction its two fused layers form the mesentery of the sigmoid colon. Where the peritoneum clothes a pelvic organ it forms an integral part of the layered structure of that organ and receives its innervation from the same nerve supply as the viscus.

The peritoneal reflection from the back of the upper part of the vagina to the anterior surface of the rectum forms a pouch of variable depth – the rectouterine pouch of Douglas – and the fused layers of peritoneum continue downwards as a thick fascia towards the perineum between the rectum and vagina – the fascia of Denonvilliers (Fig. 1.2).

Innervation of the Pelvic Viscera

The pelvic viscera are innervated by both autonomic and somatic nerves. The cord segments for sympathetic innervation are T11, 12, L1, 2, and the cord segments involved in parasympathetic supply are S2, 3, 4 (pelvic splanchnics). Segments S2 and S3 form the somatic pudendal nerve, which supplies the perineum and the terminal 2.5 cm of both the vagina and the anal canal (Fig. 1.3). Preganglionic sympathetic fibres synapse in ganglia along the major arteries of the posterior abdomen whereas the parasympathetic preganglionic fibres establish synaptic connections in ganglia close to, or in the wall of, the viscus that they supply.

Anterior Compartment, Bladder and Urethra

The bladder and urethra are innervated by a vesical plexus of sympathetic and parasympathetic nerves, each of which contains efferent (motor) and afferent (sensory) fibres. The hypogastric plexus (Fig. 1.3) also provides autonomic nerves to the bladder via the internal iliac, superior and inferior vesical and uterine arteries. Pain fibres, which are stimulated by distension, spasm, or inflammation of the bladder, run in both sympathetic (T11, 12 L1, 2) and parasympathetic (S2, 3, 4) nerves, mainly the latter.

Middle Compartment; Uterus, Fallopian Tubes, Ovaries and Vagina

The uterus and Fallopian tubes receive their autonomic nerve supply from the hypogastric plexus with branches of the uterine artery. These autonomic fibres have a common origin with those supplying the bladder. The ovaries and lateral 2 cm of the tubes receive their autonomic nerve supply from ovarian plexuses: the nerves reach the ovaries along with the ovarian arteries (Fig. 1.3). The ovarian plexuses are formed from branches of the renal, aortic and hypogastric plexuses (T11, 12, L1, 2). The upper three-quarters

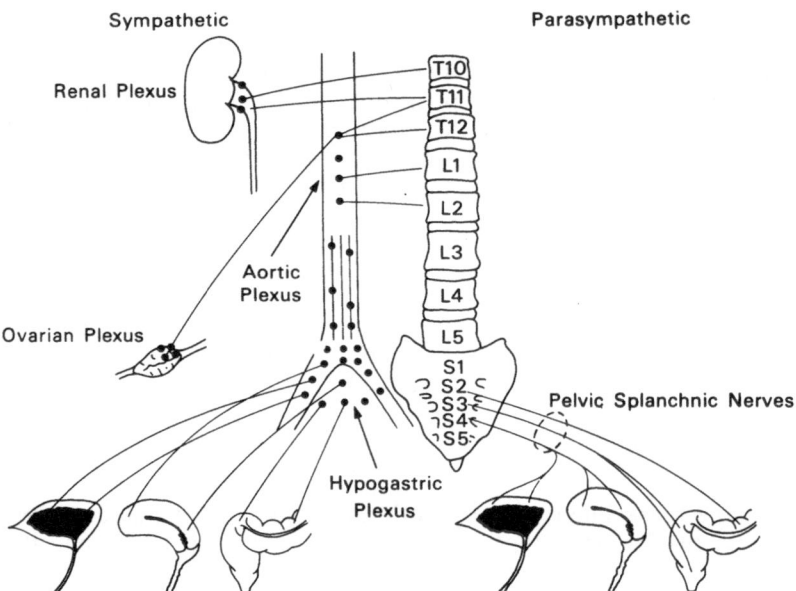

Fig. 1.3. Innervation of the pelvic viscera.

of the vagina has the same nerve supply as the uterus, whereas the distal quarter derives its supply from the pudendal nerve (S2, 3), in common with the distal 2.5 cm of the squamous portion of the anal canal.

Posterior Compartment; Rectum and Anal Canal

The rectum and upper half of the anal canal receive their vasomotor sympathetic innervation from the aortic and hypogastric plexuses along with branches of the inferior mesenteric and superior rectal (haemorrhoidal) arteries (T11, 12, L1, 2). Parasympathetic innervation is supplied by the pelvic splanchnic nerves from L2, 3, 4, which join the hypogastric plexus and are distributed to the rectum, internal half of the anal canal and internal anal sphincter muscles, together with branches of the superior and middle rectal blood vessels.

The sensory supply to the external 2.5 cm of the anal canal is from the somatic pudendal nerve (S2, 3) which, together with the perineal branch of the fourth sacral nerve (S4), innervates the external sphincter muscle (Fig. 1.3).

In view of the common sympathetic and parasympathetic innervation of the three compartments of the pelvic cavity, it is not surprising to find in clinical practice that a patient is unable to say whether visceral pain is emanating from the bladder, the genital tract or the rectum. Ancillary symptoms and physical signs will, in most instances, guide the clinician to the source of the patient's pelvic pain.

Pelvic Peritoneum

Visceral pelvic peritoneum, which covers the upper third of the bladder, the body of the uterus and the upper third of the rectum and the rectosigmoid junction, is an integral part of these organs and is innervated by autonomic nerves supplying these viscera. It is insensitive to touch but responds with pain on traction, distension, spasm or ischaemia of the viscus. Parietal pelvic peritoneum, which covers the upper half of the lateral wall of the pelvis and the upper two-thirds of the sacral hollow, is supplied by somatic nerves. These somatic nerves also supply corresponding segmental areas of skin and muscles of the trunk and anterior abdominal wall. Painful stimulation of the parietal pelvic peritoneum may cause referred segmental pain and spasm of the iliopsoas muscle and muscles of the anterior abdominal wall.

Pelvic Ureter

The abdominal ureter crosses into the pelvis at the bifurcation of the common iliac artery and is posterior to the ovary at this point. The ureter follows a course in the medial part of the broad ligament along the lateral pelvic wall towards the ischial spine and then deviates forwards and medially towards the base of the bladder, in close proximity to the uterine artery and lateral vaginal fornix. The pelvic ureter receives its autonomic nerve supply from the hypogastric plexus, which in turn is connected to the renal and aortic plexuses.

Sympathetic fibres emanate from the lower three thoracic (T10, 11, 12) and first lumbar (L1) segments of the cord and parasympathetic fibres from the second, third and fourth sacral segments (S2, 3, 4). All these fibres are thought to be mainly sensory. Distension and spasm of the ureter, e.g. by an impacted calculus, causes ureteric colic, which is referred to segmental areas T10, 11, 12, L1. The severe pain experienced by the patient starts in the loin, with radiation to the groin and labium majus. In some patients pain traverses into the upper thigh by referred radiation along the genitofemoral nerve (L1, 2).

Surgical Aspects of Female Pelvic Pain

On the basis of innervation of the pelvic organs, two types of pelvic pain are recognised — *visceral pain* due to stimulation of autonomic nerves (T11, 12, L1, 2, S2, 3, 4) and *somatic pain* due to stimulation of sensory nerve endings in the pudendal nerve (S2, 3). Pain in the female pelvis and perineum may be visceral or somatic or rarely a mixture of both. Pain in the pelvis may be acute, chronic, or referred, and, whereas this chapter highlights chronic conditions producing pain, a knowledge of acute causes of pain and their diagnosis is necessary because many of these acute conditions become chronic in due course.

Gynaecological/Obstetric Aspects of Pelvic Pain

By early adolescence the vagina, cervix and uterus have developed to functional maturity. The ovary has changed from intermittent to regular ovulation, and the menstrual cycle has started. The ovary undergoes cyclical enlargement and selective follicle maturation, culminating in the release of (usually one) ovum and minimal blood loss into the pelvic cavity some 12 to 14 days before menstruation. Retrograde menstruation through the patent Fallopian tubes may also occur. The patency of the uterine cavity and Fallopian tubes also allows infection direct access to the peritoneal cavity. These factors form a basis for peritoneal irritation, which will cause pain. There is the possibility of unilateral ovarian supremacy, but transpelvic spread of blood can produce ipsilateral, contralateral, and sometimes bilateral pain. The upper vagina is in direct contact with the lower margin of the peritoneal cavity and the pouch of Douglas and so can be sensitive to the pressure of coitus. This effect can be transmitted to adjacent organs, particularly the bladder, ovary, and rectum.

Neurophysiology of Pain

G.D. Thomas

Pain is one of the commonest reasons for medical consultation. In spite of an explosion in research and information relating to the neuroanatomy and neurophysiology of pain over the past decade, the ability to assess a patient's complaint of pain accurately remains imprecise and difficult. The following section outlines the current concepts in the anatomophysiology of pain and explains how this knowledge may be exploited.

Neuroanatomy and Physiology

Peripheral Receptors and Afferents

Nociceptive receptors, which are widespread in the tissues, detect mechanical, thermal and chemical stimuli. When the degree of stimulation becomes actually or potentially harmful (noxious), depolarisation occurs and is propagated centripetally to the neuraxis. Nociceptors have a relatively high threshold and are unaffected by stimuli that can excite the more sensitive tactile and articular mechanoreceptors.

Chemical irritation of nociceptors can be induced with a variety of agents, including lactic acid and K^+ ions (following ischaemia) and histamine, 5-hydroxytryptamine (serotonin), bradykinin and prostaglandins (following tissue damage and inflammation). Prostaglandin E_2 (PGE_2) enhances the stimulating action of bradykinin on nociceptors, thus accounting for the extreme tenderness of many inflammatory reactions. (Non-steroidal anti-inflammatory drugs act by inhibiting prostaglandin synthetase, thus reducing the concentration of PGE_2 and therefore the sensitivity of the receptors.)

The afferent fibres from the receptor system are of two types: small myelinated (A δ) fibres and (the majority) unmyelinated C fibres. This is therefore a small diameter (mostly less than 5 μm) afferent system, resulting in relatively slow conduction velocity, extreme sensitivity to local anaesthetic agents and a higher threshold to electric stimulation than fibres of larger diameter, such as mechanoreceptor afferents.

The receptors leading to the slightly faster conducting A δ fibres have lower thresholds than those leading to the unmyelinated C fibres. The A δ fibres also have a much more direct path to the thalamus, and it is these fibres which conduct the initial pinprick type stimulus which is always well localised and precedes the more diffuse information carried by the C fibres, which signal tissue injury.

Spinal Cord

On reaching the dorsal horn via posterior nerve roots, incoming impulses are subject to two important modulating influences, one segmental and the other from descending pathways from higher centres.

Segmental Mechanism. Most of the nociceptive C fibres terminate in the substantia gelatinosa of the dorsal horn. From this peripheral situation the nociceptive traffic passes centrally through different laminae before finally converging on transmission (T) cells, which are more deeply situated. The faster conducting A δ fibres have a more direct path to their transmitter cells. When sufficiently stimulated the T cell will fire, and the impulse is then conducted across the midline to ascend in the contralateral anterolateral funiculus. Low-threshold mechanoreceptor traffic travels in relatively thick myelinated fibres ascending in the dorsal columns. At their point of entry into the spinal cord, however, these fibres give off collaterals that penetrate the dorsal horn. These collaterals synapse in the deeper layers of the horn and exert an inhibitory effect on transmission between the substantia gelatinosa and the transmitter cells. When C fibre traffic is relatively light but large-fibre stimulation high, the effect of this so-called gate control mechanism is that the T cell will not be stimulated. In the reverse situation however, the T cell will fire and nociceptive information will be passed along the anterolateral tract. In conditions where large-fibre afferents become deficient, as may happen following an attack of herpes zoster, the preponderance of unopposed C fibre traffic can result in prolonged pain.

Descending Inhibitory Mechanism. Further modulation of nociceptive transmission is brought about by descending pathways from higher centres. The best described mechanism originates in the periaqueductal grey matter of the midbrain. This structure has an input of collaterals from spinothalamic axons and is particularly responsive to pinprick stimulation. Descending fibres from the periaqueductal grey matter pass along a serotoninergic pathway to the nucleus raphe magnus and then via the dorsolateral tract of the spinal cord to synapse eventually with an inhibitory interneuron. This interneuron is interpolated between the substantia gelatinosa and the nociceptive final transmitter and so is capable of blocking transmission.

Ascending Pathways. When the transmitter cell situated in the deeper laminae of the dorsal horn is sufficiently excited, it will propagate an impulse which is conveyed across the midline to ascend in the anterolateral funiculus of the spinal cord. Within this tract the fibres carrying initial or pinprick type information ascend with relatively few interruptions to the neothalamus. From here the information is relayed to the postcentral gyrus and results in accurate localisation of the pain. The fibres carrying the slightly later information of tissue injury ascend via a less direct route to the brainstem reticular formation. Some spinoreticular fibres ascend in the ipsilateral anterolateral tract, whereas others ascend independently of the main pathways. This explains why anterolateral cordotomy is not always effective in interrupting contralateral pain pathways and why its effectiveness may diminish in time. The information carried by this system is eventually relayed via the anteromedial (palaeo) thalamus to the frontal lobes, limbic system and hypothalamus. It is these connections that result in the less precise component of pain perception and the emotional response to it. The hypothalamic connection initiates the autonomic response to pain.

Visceral Pain

The viscera are innervated by the autonomic nervous system, which has sympathetic and parasympathetic components. The efferent fibres of the sympathetic system emerge through the thoracic and upper lumbar spinal nerves, and the parasympathetic efferent fibres emerge through certain cranial and sacral spinal nerves.

Viscera are insensitive to cutting, crushing or bruising. Excessive distension, contraction and pulling, however, together with some pathological conditions, excite nociceptive afferents and may result in pain. The great majority of the nociceptive afferents run within the sympathetic system. These afferents are the peripheral processes of unipolar cells situated in spinal nerve ganglia, and their courses are not interrupted by synapses in the autonomic ganglia. The sensation aroused by stimulation of these afferents is usually a poorly localised ache or, when caused by excessive contractions, colic. Occasionally, however, the pain may be referred to the same dermatome as that innervated by somatic sensory nerves which share the same vertebral inlet. The segmental inlet levels of sympathetic pelvic afferents are as follows:

Sigmoid colon and rectum	L1–2
Ureter	T11–L2
Ovary	T10–11
Urinary bladder	T11–L2
Uterus	T12–L1
Fallopian tube	T10–L1

Afferent fibres from the uterine cervix, however, are carried via the pelvic splanchnic nerves to their cells of origin in the dorsal roots of the upper sacral nerves. This explains why section of the hypogastric (presacral) plexus relieves pain in the body of the uterus but not cervical pain.

Figs. 1.3 and 1.4 illustrate the pelvic afferent pathways and the anterior abdominal dermatomes that share the same vertebral inlets.

Neuropeptides

Morphine and related strong analgesics act at specific parts of the nociceptive pathway. The densest concentration of opiate receptors is now known to be at the following sites:

Substantia gelatinosa of dorsal horn and spinal trigeminal nucleus
Ventral median raphe nuclei
Hypothalamus
Medial thalamus
Parts of limbic lobe

Enkephalins

The location of opiate receptors at strategic points along the nociceptive pathways is explained by their ability to combine with endogenously produced pain modifying substances.

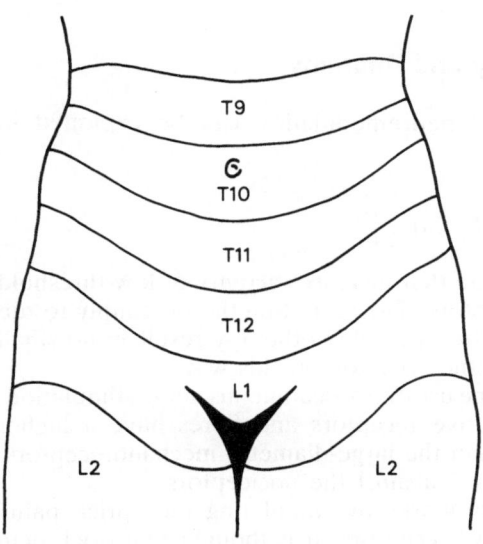

Fig. 1.4. Segmental dermatomes of anterior abdominal wall.

The first two discovered (in 1975) were termed methionine enkephalin and leucine enkephalin. Methionine enkephalin is a derivative of pituitary β-lipoprotein. β-endorphin is a longer amino-acid chain derivative of β-lipoprotein, with a longer analgesic effect.

The naturally occurring enkephalins have similar analgesic activity and side-effects to morphine, but their duration of action is very brief owing to rapid breakdown. Their actions are also opposed by naloxone. Enkephalins have been demonstrated in synaptosomal fractions of nervous tissue, suggesting a neurotransmitter role. Many neuropeptides have been discovered since 1975, the most important of which is substance P.

Substance P

Substance P has been isolated from the gut as well as nervous tissue. A high percentage of cell bodies in trigeminal and dorsal root ganglia are substance P (SP) positive, and the central processes of SP positive neurons are distributed to the substantia gelatinosa of the spinal cord. Present knowledge leads to the conclusion that SP is the neurotransmitter in primary afferents that respond to noxious stimuli. Transmission from SP containing afferents is blocked by morphine or enkephalin.

Stimulation of the periaqueductal grey matter initiates the descending inhibitory mechanism previously described leading to analgesia. Injection of morphine into the periaqueductal and adjacent grey matter produces intense analgesia.

Fig. 1.5 illustrates the likely chain of events involved in descending inhibition. When the enkephalinergic interneuron is stimulated it exerts a powerful synaptic inhibitory effect, blocking stimulation of the dorsal horn cell by SP and therefore diminishing input to the final transmitter cell (T).

Application of Neurophysiology and Anatomy

Knowledge of the mechanisms of neuromodulation can be exploited in various ways to aid pain relief.

Segmental Modulation Augmentation

This can be achieved by any method that increases activity of low-threshold tactile receptors and mechanoreceptors. The easiest method is simply to rub the affected part. The beneficial effects of physiotherapy result in no small part from the augmentation of tactile receptors in this way.

A more sophisticated method is the use of transcutaneous nerve stimulation. This utilises the fact that nociceptive receptors and fibres have a higher threshold to electric stimulation than the large-diameter mechanoreceptors, thus swinging the dorsal horn "gate" against the nociceptors.

Segmental acupuncture probably works by stimulating the "prick pain" receptors but not the "tissue injury" receptors. It is thought that prick pain

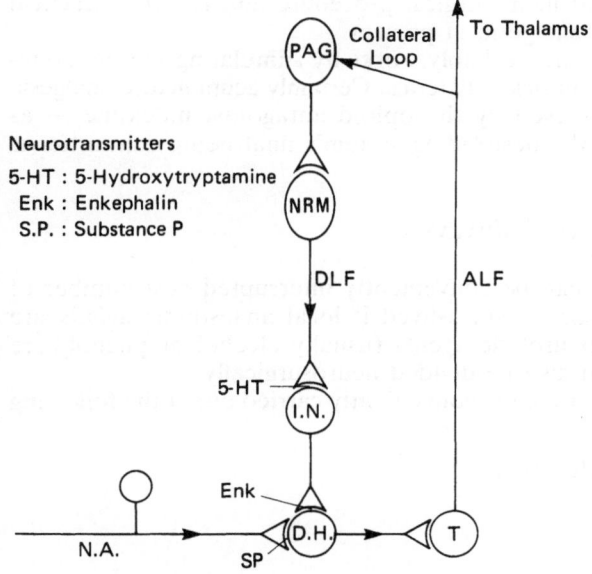

Neurotransmitters
5-HT : 5-Hydroxytryptamine
Enk : Enkephalin
S.P. : Substance P

N.A. : Nociceptive Afferent
D.H. : Dorsal Horn Neuron
T : Transmission Cell
ALF : Anterolateral Funiculus
PAG : Periaqueductal Grey Matter
NRM : Nucleus Raphe Magnus
DLF : Dorsolateral Funiculus
I.N. : Interneuron

Fig. 1.5. The chain of events involved in descending inhibition.

fibres then stimulate an inhibitory interneuron, thus blocking transmission of chronic pain carrying C fibres.

The application of cold can often be beneficial, particularly in musculo-skeletal pain, where muscle spasm is involved. This may, however, be a direct effect on the muscles involved (interrupting the cycle of pain → spasm → more pain) rather than a dorsal horn mechanism.

Similarly application of gentle warmth can be beneficial, especially in pain states secondary to nerve fibre irritation or damage.

Dorsal column stimulation is achieved by placing electrodes epidurally over the dorsal columns. Electrical stimulation of these electrodes can produce powerful analgesia in some conditions which are resistant to other methods.

Descending Inhibitory Augmentation

Descending inhibitory augmentation can be achieved by direct stimulation of the midbrain in the region of the periaqueductal grey matter. However, this is a highly complicated neurosurgical procedure and is not a practical proposition for enhancing analgesia at present.

Extrasegmental acupuncture probably works by stimulating the periaqueductal grey matter via the pinprick collaterals. Certainly acupuncture analgesia has been shown to be reversed by the opioid antagonist naloxone — as would be expected, since the descending system's final neurotransmitter is enkephalin.

Interruption of Nociceptive Pathways

The nociceptive pathways can be conveniently interrupted at a number of levels. This interruption can be short-lived if local anaesthetic agents are used or longer lasting if neurolytic agents (usually alcohol or phenol) are used. The nerve fibres can also be divided neurosurgically.

Local anaesthetic blocks are most conveniently carried out at the following sites:

Local infiltration of a tender area

Peripheral nerve block

Plexus block

Paravertebral block

Epidural injection

Intrathecal injection

For treatment of acute pain, local anaesthetic used in one of the above sites may be very effective. If the epidural route is used a catheter may be left in situ and the local anaesthetic given intermittently or by constant infusion.

For treatment of chronic pain repeated injection of local anaesthetic is sometimes surprisingly effective. In planning analgesia for intractable pain, the effect of a local anaesthetic block may be a useful predictor of the effectiveness of a planned neurolytic procedure.

Neurolytic injections for somatic pain are now carried out infrequently because epidural opiate injection is more effective. However, the technique still has a place where very severe pain is limited to one or two dermatomes. The most effective route is intrathecal.

The classic neurosurgical technique for intractable pain relief is anterolateral cordotomy. This procedure results in contralateral loss of pain and temperature sensation below the level of the lesion and is used for severe unilateral pain that cannot be otherwise controlled. The beneficial effect of this procedure may wear off after 9 months or so, so it should be reserved for those patients with a relatively short survival expectation.

Neurolytic block of peripheral somatic nerves sometimes results in a subsequent neuritis, so this technique is not now used. Freezing a peripheral nerve with a cryoprobe will, however, produce a much longer interruption of sensory conduction than local anaesthesia and has a very low incidence of neuritis, so is often worth considering, particularly for chronic benign pain.

Sympathetic Block

Visceral pain is transmitted via the sympathetic afferents. It follows, therefore, that interruption of sympathetic fibres will contribute effectively to pain control where visceral pathology is involved. Sympathetic blocks are most conveniently carried out at the following sites:

Lumbar paravertebral
Coeliac plexus
Stellate ganglion.

Neurolytic block of the coeliac plexus is particularly helpful for upper abdominal malignancies. For pelvic visceral pain the exact route of the fibres involved can never be accurately known, particularly if the pain is in the midline. In unilateral pelvic malignant pain, a trial local anaesthetic lumbar sympathetic block may be tried and, if successful, followed by neurolytic block. In general, however, sympathetic block is not as successful for pelvic pain as it is for coeliac axis pain.

Epidural Opiates

Since the substantia gelatinosa of the dorsal horn is rich in opiate receptors it should follow that locally introduced opiates would produce intense analgesia. This has been found to be so: subarachnoid injection of morphine 0.5 to 1 mg will produce relief for up to 24 hours from the severe pain of infiltrating malignancies. Subsequently it was found that epidural injection of rather higher doses (2 to 5 mg) resulted in equally good but shorter lived analgesia. The disadvantage of this technique is the risk of respiratory depression, which is higher in subarachnoid than epidural administration. The highly lipid soluble fentanyl and diamorphine have a more rapid and more localised effect than the poorly soluble morphine; and because a higher percentage is absorbed, less is available for rostral spread in the cerebrospinal fluid. Because of the ever present possibility of respiratory depression, however, patients given this type of analgesia for acute pain should be nursed in high dependency units. Patients with intractable malignant pain, however, who will already be taking high doses of opiates by other routes, develop a high degree of resistance to the respiratory depressant effect of opiates and in most cases can be managed at home after stabilisation in hospital.

Psychological Aspects of Pelvic Pain

J. M. Hughes

Psychosomatic Medicine

In the 1920s and 1930s psychosomatic medicine tended to concentrate on the psychoanalysis of individual patients and on relating a particular personality profile to a specific illness. Neither concept has stood the tests of time or of scientific analysis.

Modern workers have emphasised that all illness has a psychological component and that in many illnesses it is the joint effect of psychosocial and physical causes that produces the presenting illness. Constitutional factors are also seen as important, as demonstrated by family, twin and adoption studies. There is often some inherent sensitivity of the target organ – a sensitivity that may originate in both physical and psychological happenings in the patient's past life.

The Psychology of Pain

Psychological factors have powerful influences on the feeling of pain. An individual's threshold of pain is fairly constant and has a mainly physiological basis. It is not greatly influenced by psychological factors. However, an individual's pain tolerance is heavily influenced by psychological factors. It can be increased by reducing anxiety, by distraction and by motivation.

How an individual reacts to and expresses pain is influenced by both cultural and individual backgrounds. For some, ethnic and family backgrounds can profoundly affect complaints of pain. In others, the personality make-up is the important influence, the expression of pain being closely related to the degree of extraversion. Pain is felt more acutely by anxious patients.

Complaints of pain are highly correlated with the degree of neuroticism shown by an individual. They can be broadly of two types:

1. Tension pain – a reaction to frightening stress, especially if it is long drawn out.
2. Conversion pain – where a conflict in a patient's life is converted into a physical symptom which reflects the underlying unresolved conflict and affects the individual's feeling of wellbeing.

Personality profiles of outpatients with chronic pain fall into an intermediate position between those of psychiatric patients on the one hand and those of patients with "straightforward" physical illness on the other. However, patients with predominantly organic illness have high scores for neurosis if the pain is long drawn out. Acute pain tends to be associated with feelings of anxiety but not with a neurotic personality profile. Chronic pain can lead to emotional disturbance expressed as a neurotic presentation very similar to that seen in functional pain.

Pelvic Pain in Women

This common symptom presents special difficulties in assessment. In addition to psychological influences, there are many pelvic body systems that can malfunction. It is an area where a number of medical disciplines meet. Cooperation is essential to accurate diagnosis. It is important that all involved try to speak with one voice to the patient.

The pelvis has symbolic importance for women, and this is particularly important in relation to sexual function, to reproduction and in marital relationships. Doctors must be sensitive to this aspect of pelvic disease, which is seldom articulated by the patient in words. In many cases, a combined physical and psychological approach is needed.

Psychogenic pain has some well-defined characteristics. It is often ill-defined, and its anatomical distribution depends more on the patient's concepts than on clinical disease processes. Such pain often does not radiate, commonly the patient presents with multiple unrelated symptoms, and the fluctuations in the course of the illness are determined more by crises in the patients's psychosocial life than by physical changes.

There are usually well-defined personality and social histories of the type found in maladjusted patients. The patient is likely to have had many previous hospital admissions – not necessarily to psychiatric hospitals. Many features have been described in the personality make-up of such patients. They are usually in the age range 20–40 and have difficulty in accepting a feminine role. Many have difficulty, too, in expressing anger and in achieving independence as an individual. They are more responsive to a psychological approach and their personality profiles (e.g. the Minnesota Multiphasic Personality Inventory) show high scores on hysteria and hypochondriasis.

Psychological Investigation of Chronic Pelvic Pain

A psychological component should always be added to the investigation of chronic pelvic pain in women. In exploring the psychosocial background, the doctor needs sensitive antennae to pick up those messages that the patient is unlikely to verbalise.

A careful unhurried assessment of the psychological organic balance of causation is needed. It should not usually be necessary to refer such a patient to a psychiatrist; indeed, there are real advantages in such an assessment being carried out by the gynaecologist who has already built up a relationship with the patient.

It is important to recognise that substantial psychopathology is likely to be present irrespective of the physical findings. In patients with chronic pain, psychological profiles do not distinguish those with organic pathology from those without such pathology. By contrast, patients with chronic pelvic disorders but without pain show more normal personality profiles. Social class is not relevant. Specific psychiatric illnesses can occur in this setting and would normally suggest referral for psychiatric treatment. Such conditions include:

1. Neurosis, including conversion hysteria (the commonest finding).
2. Severe depression, which can present with apparent organic type pain.
3. Schizophrenia. The clue is the patient's description of and preoccupation with the pain, to the extent that it can be delusional.
4. Obsessional disorders. Patients who may be too rigid to be able to adjust to changes in their bodies.

Therapeutic Implications

The psychological approach used will depend on the underlying pathology and the patient's personality.

1. Patients with substantial pelvic pathology vary in personality, and the more vulnerable need greater attention to their psychological needs.
2. If the pelvic pathology is insufficient to account for the symptoms a more detailed psychological assessment is needed.
3. In patients with minor physical findings or no pathology a more obviously neurotic personality is likely – perhaps even conversion/hysteria. Psychological treatment is more important, and the help of a psychiatrist may be needed.
4. Patients with chronic pain inevitably develop more and more hypochondriacal attitudes, and the doctor must modify his approach to the patient accordingly.

The first step in psychological treatment lies in an investigation of the patient's development and background. Particular attention should be paid to the childhood environment and the relationship with the parents. Marital relations are of great importance, as is the sexual history, with special emphasis on the patient's adjustment to sexual life. The patient should be asked whether she has had a history of psychiatric illness, but this should be done tactfully in a patient who considers her illness to be physically based.

The building up of a different doctor/patient relationship as a result of such an approach is a powerful treatment in itself.

There may be the need for formal specialist psychiatric treatment, which could be broadly psychotherapeutic or based on physical treatments, mainly with psychoactive drugs.

In chronic illness of this sort, surgical intervention should be approached cautiously. In many cases the patient presses for what she sees as an answer to her problem.

Some Specific Conditions

Dysmenorrhoea. In primary dysmenorrhoea, physiological causes are all-important, although the actual presentation of symptoms may be influenced by psychological factors.

Premenstrual Tension. There are important cyclical physical changes in the pelvis and in the body generally. Nevertheless, the psychology of the patient is important. Complaints of irritability, tension and depression are often an exaggeration of the patient's normal personality and are more likely to occur in those with obsessional or hysterical personalities.

Dyspareunia. There are many causes, both physical and psychological, for dyspareunia. In non-organic cases, lack of lubrication is the basic cause.

This can occur for many reasons: poor sexual technique, fear of intercourse, fear of pregnancy, a poor marital relationship, distaste for sex, and psychiatric syndromes. These patients need an educational approach as well as psychotherapeutically based treatment.

Vaginismus. In vaginismus psychogenic factors are paramount. Such patients show similar psychopathology to those with dyspareunia – lack of sexual experience, emotional unpreparedness, fear of coitus and, commonly, distaste for sex. These patients need education about sex and psychotherapeutic treatment directed at the reasons for their poor sexual adjustment. Physical measures are needed too – self-exploration to help overcome misconceptions about their bodies, combined with the use of serial dilators and, if necessary, with instruction in relaxation techniques. The involvement of the sexual partner in the treatment process may be vital.

Chronic Pelvic Pain without Obvious Pathology. Psychological factors are important in such patients but not necessarily causative. These patients constitute a diagnostic rag bag that calls for extensive investigation, both physically and psychologically. Emotional symptoms are intense and occur whether the pain is organic or non-organic. This can be an area where emotional interactions with the doctor occur. It is very easy for such patients to feel that the doctor does not understand them or is unsympathetic. Combined treatment from a gynaecologist, a psychiatrist and a "pain" doctor may be needed.

Anxiety of Referral

Seeing a doctor is for most people a stressful event. Before settling down to the technicalities of the consultation it is worth devoting a few minutes to a general discussion aimed at putting the patient at ease and at raising her confidence. The doctor/patient relationship is in itself a powerful therapeutic tool.

Special care is needed with patients with chronic illness. They are often experienced observers of doctors. Commonly they are disillusioned, believing that the doctor will not believe them or will be unable to help them. Doctors commonly give a sigh of frustration when such a patient appears in a busy clinic with a seemingly interminable history and a bulging case file. It is important to make a fresh approach to the patient's problems with an open mind.

The Approach to Cancer and Cancerophobia

The Patient with Cancer

The psychological approach to cancer patients is an important and sometimes neglected subject. Despite the improved prognosis today for some forms of cancer, it is still a diagnosis that strikes terror in many hearts. Significantly, cancer patients have a higher than average suicide rate.

In the search for the most effective physical approaches, we should not neglect the patient's emotional reactions to the diagnosis of cancer. There are some general principles worth following. Honesty is the best policy, but delivering the bad news calls for special skills and a carefully worked out approach. A minority of patients cannot face the truth, and there should always be an exploratory discussion to determine whether the patient belongs to this minority. If she does she should not be told.

Follow-up discussions with both the patient and her family are essential. Discussion with other caring staff, especially nurses, should be routine, not only to support those staff in a demanding role but also to ensure that all staff give broadly the same message to the patient.

For patients who are dying the same principles apply, perhaps in an intensified way. Certainly most patients cope better when they know the facts.

Cancerophobia

Cancerophobia is a symptom and not a diagnosis. It can occur in a variety of psychiatric settings.

1. Cancerophobia can occur as part of a phobic (neurotic) illness but is less common than agoraphobia, social phobias etc. The treatment is that of the neurosis and is largely psychological – either the traditional psychotherapeutic approach or a behavioural approach or a combination of the two.

2. Cancerophobia is a common symptom in severe depression. Depression usually responds well to treatment, and with it the fear of cancer. Treatment should be largely physical, i.e. with antidepressant drugs or infrequently with electroconvulsive therapy. The alert doctor should always be on the lookout for hidden depression behind the presenting symptoms. The diagnosis can usually be established without great difficulty by investigating the patient's mood.

3. Cancerophobia is a rare presenting symptom in schizophrenia. The experienced observer has a clue from the totally unrealistic way in which the patient describes the symptom, raising it to the level of a delusion. One must always have supporting evidence before making such a serious diagnosis.

4. The term cancerophobia should not be applied to a patient reasonably asking for reassurance that she does not have cancer.

Standard Drugs used in Psychiatry

Anxiolytics

Benzodiazepine anxiolytics have fallen under a cloud recently as a consequence of the development of widespread dependence in the Western world. The preferred approach to patients with neurosis is a psychotherapeutic one based on counselling aided by anxiety reducing techniques such as relaxation training sessions. Benzodiazepines should be used sparingly and normally not for more than 3 to 4 weeks.

Example: diazepam 5–10 mg bd or tds.

Night Sedation

Hypnotics should be avoided as far as possible. If prescribed, using the drug on alternate nights only can make dependence less likely. Long-term prescribing should be resisted.

Example: temazepam 10–20 mg at night.

Drugs with a longer half-life, such as nitrazepam, should not be used in patients aged over 65.

Antidepressants

There are a large number of antidepressant drugs with comparatively little difference in their efficacy. All have side-effects (e.g. dry mouth, constipation), which are mostly a nuisance rather than serious.

There are two main groups of antidepressants:

tricyclic and quadricyclic drugs
monoamine oxidase inhibitors (MAOIs), which are specially effective in depression accompanied by phobic and other neurotic symptoms.

A sufficient dose must be given, and treatment should be continued for 3 to 6 months. The dose of drug should be reduced progressively when the patient has been back to normal for a month.

Examples:
clomipramine (a tricyclic) 75–150 mg daily in divided doses with the biggest dose at night
tranylcypromine (MAOI) 10 mg tds.

Patients taking MAOIs must avoid foods containing tyramine. An explanatory card is given to each patient with the drug.

Prophylactic Drugs

Both lithium and carbamazepine are effective preventatives in patients with chronic disturbances of mood, whether presenting with mania or depression. The treatment must be carefully monitored with regular estimations of the serum lithium level.

Examples:
lithium carbonate 250–500 mg bd
carbamazepine 400–800 mg daily.

Drugs in Schizophrenia

The major tranquillisers (antischizophrenic drugs) have limited relevance to pelvic pain in women. They are effective in controlling many of the more disturbing symptoms of psychosis, including thought disorder and behavioural disturbance. Where longer-term treatment is necessary consideration should be given to using the drug in a depot injection form. The advantages include a smaller daily dose of drug and a reduced "drop out" rate from treatment.

Examples:

chlorpromazine 50 mg tds.

trifluoperazine 5–10 mg bd.

depot injections:
    fluphenazine decanoate 25–50 mg I M monthly.
    flupenthixol decanoate 20–60 mg I M monthly.

If neurological side-effects occur an antiparkinsonian agent should also be given, e.g. benzhexol 5 mg bd or tds.

Warning

Patients taking psychotropic drugs should be warned not to drive if they feel drowsy. Alcohol should be avoided.

2 Examination and Investigation

E.J.G. GLENCROSS, A. JONES, D.G. JONES,
I. ROCKER and D.E. STURDY

General and Surgical Examination

D. E. Sturdy

In general surgical practice about 60 % of patients with chronic pelvic pain will be direct referrals, 30 % will have been referred by gynaecologists and fewer than 10 % will have been seen by an orthopaedic surgeon. Nearly all the patients with acute and chronic perineal disorders will have been referred directly to the general surgical clinic. The surgeon will need to ascertain, by detailed history taking and physical examination, the most probable source of the patient's pain and to allocate the symptoms and signs to one compartment of the pelvic cavity. The patient will be referred to an orthopaedic surgeon or gynaecologist as appropriate. If the patient has been referred from a gynaecologist she will have had a pelvic examination and probably a pelvic ultrasound or computed tomographic scan. Patients referred from the orthopaedic department will have had a straight X-ray of the abdomen and pelvis.

The presentation of lower abdominal pain in women is related to age (Table 2.1). Both acute and chronic conditions occur from early adulthood to a few years past the menopause, and whereas this is a very broad grouping it nevertheless illustrates the importance of sexuality, pregnancy, endometriosis and the group for which no obvious pathology is detected and which are placed under the heading of gynaecalgia.

Examination for Acute Painful Conditions of the Perineum

The diagnosis of painful lesions of the perineum is visual. For complete examination the patient will need to be in the lithotomy position, since the external anterior (urinary) and the middle (genital) compartments of the pelvis cannot be adequately inspected in any other way. A urethral caruncle will be exposed by gentle separation of the labia. If the patient has a

Table 2.1. Age related lower abdominal/pelvic pain

	< Puberty	Adolescence	20–39	40–55	56+
Sexual assault					
Incest					
STD/PID					
Dyspareunia					
1° dysmenorrhoea					
2° dysmenorrhoea					
Premenstrual tension					
Ovarian cysts					
Pregnancy					
Uterus					
Endometriosis					
Prolapse					
Surgical					
Urological					
Psychogenic					
"Gynaecalgia"					

PID, pelvic inflammatory disease; STD, sexually transmitted disease.

Bartholin's abscess the affected labium majus will be oedematous, swollen and tender to palpation, and in these circumstances vaginal examination should not be attempted. Painful lesions of the posterior (rectal) compartment will be readily visible. Thrombosed external piles, anal fissures, strangulated piles and perianal and ischiorectal abscesses are all extremely painful, and digital examination of the rectum is inadvisable. The clinician must make certain that when these painful conditions have resolved on treatment a full examination of the rectum and sigmoid colon, as outlined below, is undertaken to exclude disease of the lower bowel.

Examination for Acute Pelvic Pain

In the diagnosis of acute pelvic inflammatory disease both vaginal and rectal examination are mandatory. Tenderness and pain within the pelvis on pressure over the cervix indicates pelvic peritoneal inflammation, possibly due to acute appendicitis, salpingitis or diverticulitis. Similarly pelvic inflammatory masses due to Crohn's disease of the ileum, diverticular disease of the sigmoid colon and salingo-ovarian masses may be palpable bimanually, occasionally with difficulty if the patient is resistant. Many pelvic inflammatory conditions produce a pelvic abscess, palpable rectally as a tender boggy mass in the anterior rectal wall which indents on digital pressure. This examination is undoubtedly extremely uncomfortable but produces information of exceptional diagnostic value.

Examination for Chronic Pelvic Pain

Evaluation of Symptoms

In an attempt to compartmentalise the patient's symptoms a detailed history is essential. Information about the pain needs to be elicited as follows:

Duration; type of onset; periodicity

Characteristics (colicky, dragging, sharp, stabbing)

Relation to posture or movement, menses, micturition or defaecation

Whether relieved by analgesics or other medication.

Ancillary evaluation of urinary compartment symptoms includes specific questions about bladder function – frequency, dysuria, haematuria, suprapubic discomfort, difficulty in passing urine and pneumaturia. The features of haematuria are a valuable guide to diagnosis.

Blood at beginning of micturition indicates urethral or bladder neck origin.

Blood at end of micturition indicates possible ureteric origin.

Bright red blood mixed throughout urine sample and absence of pain suggests bladder neoplasm.

Dark red blood mixed throughout urine sample in bladder infection.

Large fleshy clots in bloody urine indicate bladder carcinoma or cystitis.

Spindle shaped clots in pink urine are ureteric clots.

Ancillary evaluation of rectal compartment symptoms is based on questioning about:

Bowel frequency (diarrhoea or constipation)

Change in bowel habit

Blood in stools

Mucus in stools

Anal discharge (faeces, blood, mucus or pus)

Feeling of something "coming down the canal"

Feeling of swelling around anal orifice

Feeling of incomplete defaecation

Explosive defaecation – flatus plus liquid motions

The diagnostic significance of blood in stools depends on whether it is:

Smeared on stool surface (piles or anal carcinoma)

Mixed with motions (inflammatory bowel disease or carcinoma)

Passed separately from motion (carcinoma of rectum)

Splashed around toilet pan (haemorrhoids)

The colour of blood is also important:

Bright red indicates a lower rectal source (usually piles)

Pink indicates inflammatory bowel disease

Dark red originates in the upper rectum or sigmoid colon (carcinoma of rectosigmoid)

Black (melaena) indicates bleeding from upper gastrointestinal tract (stomach or duodenum).

Previous history should include details of previous serious illnesses and, in particular, abdominal or pelvic operations or radiotherapy treatment. A family history of urinary or bowel disease, e.g. familial polyposis, is also important.

Armed with the information obtained from these questions the surgeon should be able to estimate the probable source of the patient's pain and to proceed to a detailed physical examination with a specific pelvic compartment in mind.

Clinical Examination

For a complete examination of the pelvis the abdomen and lower limbs are fully exposed. A visual inspection of the patient in both prone and supine positions is undertaken, the surgeon looking specifically for swelling or distension of the lower abdomen, the presence of a femoral or inguinal bulge, swelling or oedema of the lower limbs and swelling over the sacrum or gluteal areas. The abdomen is systematically palpated, with special reference to masses arising from the pelvis, dull to percussion and palpated in the hypogastrium. The distended bladder is palpable in the midline in the hypogastric area and is dull to percussion.

The inguinal and iliac regions are examined for evidence of inguinal lymphadenopathy, and the inguinal and femoral orifices are palpated for a cough impulse or evidence of herniation. The femoral pulses are identified on each side, and the arteries are auscultated for bruits. The patient is next examined in the lithotomy position with a thorough inspection of the perineum for evidence of caruncles, fissures, fistulae and, rarely, neoplastic condition in the anal canal. In the lithotomy position a bimanual examination of the pelvis is undertaken (p. 00) for evidence of disease of the vagina and cervix or of tumours and masses within the pelvic cavity.

Rectal Examination

Further examination concentrates on the posterior (colorectal) pelvic compartment. The patient is placed on the left lateral position (for a right handed surgeon), and a lubricated right index finger is inserted into the rectum for thorough palpation of all quadrants of the rectal ampulla. The uterine cervix is nearly always palpable anteriorly, outside the rectal wall, and so are ring pessaries and occasionally intrauterine devices. In the normal rectum the mucosa is smooth and moves freely over surrounding structures. With the rectal finger in position the patient is asked to strain slightly, as if to attempt passage of a stool, and by this means the rectosigmoid junction may descend on to the tip of the palpating finger. Quite frequently, at this stage of the examination, globular masses about 2 cm in diameter may be palpable through the rectal wall. These masses can be identified as faeces in the sigmoid colon by gentle pressure with the fingertip, which causes indentation of the excreta. On withdrawal of the finger the glove is closely inspected for blood or mucus. A Clinistix method of examination for blood is available in all clinics.

Proctoscopy and Rectosigmoidoscopy

A well-lubricated proctoscope inserted into the anal canal gives a clear view of the anal canal and pile-bearing area. The proctoscope hardly ever demonstrates the rectum itself.

Rectosigmoidoscopy should always be preceded by digital examination of the rectum. Two types of sigmoidoscope are available – a rigid scope 25 cm long and a flexiscope 35 cm long. With practice, either of these instruments can be negotiated through the rectosigmoid junction into the sigmoid colon. It is important that this examination is undertaken in a conscious patient, because anal sphincteric control is necessary to contain the air introduced under pressure to distend the lower bowel. Biopsies of suspicious areas in the bowel are taken at this examination. Some surgeons prefer a knee–elbow position for examination of the terminal large bowel, but this is unnecessary and somewhat degrading for the patient.

Cystoscopy

If further examination of the anterior (urinary) compartment is necessary a flexiscope may be used in the female as an outpatient procedure. A cystoscopy in the female is relatively painless and is merely uncomfortable during bladder distension. Bladder examination with a flexiscope serves to exclude pathology in the urinary bladder.

Urinalysis

In the outpatient clinic a freshly passed midstream urinary sample is examined for abnormal coloration or abnormal constituents or deposit. The sample of urine is divided into two portions – one for microscopical examination and culture and the other for cytology (p. 31).

Inpatient examination

After investigation in the clinic there will remain a small group of patients in whom a positive diagnosis cannot be made and in a few patients many of these outpatient investigations are not possible because of lack of cooperation, obesity or fixation of the hip joints. In this group (under 15 %) hospital admission may be necessary to achieve a positive diagnosis. In combination with a gynaecologist the patient will be examined under an anaesthetic, and in most instances laparoscopy, cystoscopy and sigmoidoscopy will be carried out at the same time.

If a sigmoidoscopy has been unrewarding the patient may undergo colonoscopy under sedation. After adequate bowel preparation an expert colonoscopist is able to examine the whole of the large bowel, as far as the caecum in many instances. Biopsies of the bowel are obtained during colonoscopy, and colonic polyps can be removed by diathermy excision during this procedure.

Gynaecological Examination and Investigation

I. Rocker

Gynaecological History

Despite pressure on time a good rapport can be established with the patient and the necessary information elicited if the history taking is structured. Whether a prepared questionnaire is used or a factual record made depends on personal preference. The latter can be developed according to the "feel" of the interview. Each symptom sub-group is then structured to discover which symptoms are disturbing the patient and what pathological change may be present.

The presenting symptom is not always the key to understanding, since it may simply be the patient's means of requesting help, the pain complained of being an indicator of distress rather than arising from pathological change. It is therefore helpful to guide the consultation to provide indications of social circumstance, wider family responsibility, occupation in addition to housework and motherhood and particularly the advice and the comments that may have been proffered by friends and family. We are all aware of the anxiety induced by a recollection of someone with lower abdominal pains later being discovered to have advanced ovarian carcinoma. If such anxiety is not highlighted then subsequent discussion and investigation may not pay direct attention to this particular concern. The understandable anxiety of the population to cancer risk and the knowledge that there are some cancer prone families should ensure that such facts be elicited. The obstetric history should pay attention to family experience in addition to the routine information of timing of pregnancy, duration of pregnancy, health during pregnancy, foetal outcome and fulfilment of fertility wish. Past obstetric tragedy is often not discussed within a family circle. If there is a possibility of inherited disease, the wider family experience will be an indicator of anxiety.

The menstrual history is often considered to be the easiest to obtain, but at secondary consultation many patients will give a different account of the history of presentation and particularly of the sequence and the duration of blood loss. Except for those women who keep a menstrual calendar, regularity has a wide definition. There is a considerable variation of personal menstrual experience and therefore it is the change that requires analysis. The blood loss is usually well described except at the extremes of pinky discharge or the black of old altered blood. Changes such as blood clotting and profuse sudden bleeding causing embarrassment are accurate, but it is advisable to check that it is not the actual loss which is the concern but the fear that the blood loss will cause embarrassment. Normal menstrual loss is less than 60 ml in 4 to 5 days and requires an average of four tampons or pads per day. Estimation of volume loss is difficult. More than 15 ml per day may be lost before the regenerative power of the haemopoietic system is overtaken and significant anaemia develops.

Painful menstruation needs demarcation in relation to the exact time of onset, its duration in relation to the actual days of menstrual loss and also some assessment of resentment. A teenager will commonly attend with her mother, but it is advisable to allow the youngster to give her own history on her own, if necessary.

The family history of maternal or sibling painful menstruation should be recorded, as should childhood discomfort of "abdominal migraine". Some insight into the education and preparation for menstruation often gives a guideline as to sexual fantasy and as to whether there has been any possibility of sexual abuse in childhood. There is some evidence that the latter is associated with subsequent pelvic pain. The onset of menstruation in 95 % of women is between 11 and 15 years of age. Breast development takes place from approximately 9 years of age and may not be completed until pregnancy. In approximately 5 %, however, breast development is rapid and is an indication of precocious puberty, particularly if the secondary sexual characteristics have started before age 9 and are associated with the onset of menstruation. It is also important to determine whether there has been any history of diethylstilboestrol exposure in utero.

Women of all ages are remarkably frank in giving an indication of their sexual life. The relationship of sexual experience and pelvic pain relies on a careful discussion aimed on giving the patient confidence. The majority of patients will enter into discussion given the opportunity to do so, if the timing of the question is carefully chosen or even delayed for a second interview and the possibility given of choice of the sex of the interviewer.

Patients whose sexually related pain is due to underlying vaginal or pelvic pathology will usually give a direct history of their difficulties. Problems arise with those who only give an indirect intimation of a sexual problem under the symptom of pain. Inexperience, unfulfilled sexual expectation, fear of pregnancy, previous sexual trauma or rape may be presented as primary vaginismus or pelvic pain. The most difficult subgroup is those in whom a psychosexual problem is suspected but with whom discussion does not ensue. It is then that history taking becomes most important, and this may only be possible after a number of interviews have engendered mutual respect and rapport.

The bladder, small bowel, sigmoid and rectum may be affected by gynaecological disease, and the response will be in relation to the pressure or displacement of these organs by direct swelling, by reaction to an adjacent infection or the spill of blood, menstrual fluid or infected material. In the case of the bladder, this will produce frequency of micturition both day and night and urgency without dysuria. Similarly, bowel symptoms may be those of altered or alternating habit rather than persistent symptoms and therefore differentiation into primary and secondary effect is necessary.

Gynaecological Examination

The abdominal examination follows standard general principles with the guidelines of detection of change in the pelvic organs. Inspection in a good light is mandatory and if undertaken on a bed or low settee the patient should be moved to its firm edge. Modern laparoscopic or small transverse lower abdominal incisions are easily missed but are of particular significance in cases where previous chronic pelvic inflammatory disease is suspected. Asking the patient to explain such scars needs to be done delicately if the husband or a chaperone is present. Many patients are anxious about examination, and closed eyes should warn the doctor to palpate the abdomen very gently. Deep breathing to relax the abdomen is not very helpful, as it can induce overbreathing and rarely a tetanic reaction. One or two breaths to allow deeper palpation on expiration are very useful. Raising the head and shoulders to elicit tenderness in the recti can help in reaching a decision as to whether the cause for tenderness is intramuscular or intraperitoneal. Auscultation and percussion in the absence of abdominal swelling is not particularly helpful. The palpation of a swelling can outline its shape and guide its anterior and lateral extent and its texture. The latter should not be considered as absolutely diagnostic, because a cystic fibroid or a tense ovarian cyst can feel remarkably similar, particularly when there is an adipose blanket.

Pelvic Examination

No position is ideal for the inspection and bimanual examination of the pelvic organs. In domiciliary practice the basic problems that may make an examination unreliable are lack of a good light source and that the standard

Table 2.2. Pelvic examination

	Dorsal	Lithotomy	Left lateral	Sims'
Cost	+	+++	+	+
Assistance	±	++	++	+
Vision	+	+++	+	++
Compliance	+++	+	++	++

bed or divan is low and usually sags in its centre. Table 2.2 outlines the four main positions, and each has its advocate for the prime position for examination. The left lateral and Sims' have very similar advantages and are best used when examination has to be undertaken in a hospital bed or at home, as it will allow the posterior buttock to project to the edge of the bed. The left lateral will require assistance to support the anterior leg. Both positions are associated with good patient compliance, and many feel that the palpation of the posterior fornix is superior. They are therefore good positions for home examination. The dorsal and lithotomy positions allow a similar range of examination. Both need a firm base or couch for examination, but the dorsal position does not have the disadvantage of having to put the patient in lithotomy poles. The dorsal position is not suitable for the assessment of lesser degrees of prolapse, and there can also be problems in vaginal visualisation if the patient is obese or has a deficient perineum, which causes the vaginal orifice to point downwards. The lithotomy position is best for both inspection and palpation but requires assistance and either an adapted standard couch or a specially designed lithotomy chair. It is also the best position for intravaginal or intrauterine manipulation such as the placement of a coil. It does, however, worry some patients, who tend to feel isolated because their legs are hanging in stirrups. It is important to obtain experience with all positions, although the majority of examinations will be undertaken in one particular position. The question of which is best is open to discussion, the best guide being one's own experience.

It is standard teaching that vaginal examination should be performed with the well-lubricated first two fingers of the right hand. The modern good-quality plastic disposable glove does not require a lubricant unless the vagina is abnormally dry. Lubrication can invalidate cytological and bacteriological specimens taken immediately after digital examination and can also cause discomfort if it exudes on to the patient's labia and then on to her underwear. Thicker gloves on both hands are advisable in infective risk situations. The labia should be parted with the forefinger alone, first touching the introitus and then being introduced into the vagina: with experience it is not always necessary to introduce a second finger. If this is required, gentle depression of the perineum will allow easy access of the second finger. The dorsal position produces some limitation of access to the pouch of Douglas, which can be overcome by secondary rectal examination. The lithotomy position allows much deeper palpation of the pelvis and the contents of the pouch of Douglas. The lateral position also allows full examination of the pouch of Douglas, which is greater on the right side of the pelvis if the patient is lying on her left side. For a domiciliary consultation, the Sims' position on the edge of the bed is preferable, but for the consulting room either the dorsal or the left lateral, as one will have the assistance of a nurse, but for full examination, and particularly if any associated minor operative procedure is to be undertaken, the lithotomy position is the best. Only experience will tell whether a pelvic examination is sufficiently complete.

Systematic inspection of the vulva and of the introitus is undertaken. Bimanual examination is then carried out to assess the size, site, relationship, texture, mobility and tenderness of the normal pelvic organs and any palpable anomalies. The positions of the uterus and cervix are not usually difficult to assess because of their continuity and combined mobility. In the presence of acute retroflexion, enlargement of the uterus with or without fibroids can produce difficulties, e.g., a retroverted uterus may appear to be larger than it actually is. Moving both the abdominal and vaginal hands at the same time can also confuse the palpation. It is preferable to keep each hand still in turn. Alternatively both hands can be kept still, the patient asked to take a few slow deep breaths and palpation carried out during the expiratory movement, which allows deeper penetration.

Whilst the margins of the bony pelvis are readily felt and can be accurately measured, the apparent size of the uterus is sometimes misleading, particularly in the posterior part of the pelvis, so that the body of the retroverted, retroflexed uterus feels bigger in that position than when it is anteverted. It is helpful to use linear measurement to describe size. The uterus is 2.5 cm $\times$ 5 cm $\times$ 7.5 cm and the pelvis approximately 10–12 cm in diameter. The sacral promontory is rarely palpable but is usually some 10 cm from the undersurface of the symphysis pubis. The most common abnormalities are nodules, either single or multiple, or swellings of variable size and texture and are either part of or attached to the uterus, Fallopian tubes, ovaries or pelvic peritoneum. Less commonly the lower bowel and rarely bone or other retroperitoneal structures are of abnormal configuration. The relevance of pain and tenderness elicited by examination is the result of experience and awareness of the shortcomings of a particular examination. A single finger intravaginally and the use of deep expiration for palpation enables a gentle examination to be undertaken.

Examination with a bivalve speculum allows excellent inspection of the cervix and the vault of the vagina. It is deficient in visualising the anterior wall of the vagina and may mask the minor degrees of prolapse. This type of speculum can be used in either the lateral or the dorsal position. Sims' speculum is useful for the left lateral or the semiprone position, but for direct inspection of the cervix, a bivalve speculum is preferable.

Orthopaedic Examination

D. G. Jones

The orthopaedic examination of women with pelvic pain is based on a good clinical history, with particular note of any motion-related or postural pain. On examination it is important to watch mobility to see whether there is any lumbar scoliosis that might be causing nerve root entrapment or any obvious Trendelenberg limp. Lumbar spine movement should then be assessed, particular attention being paid to restriction or tilt in forward flexion indicative of lumbar root irritation. Lumbar rotation should give an estimate of sacroiliac pain, and straight-leg raising should exclude any significant root entrapment. It is important to examine the more proximal lumbar and distal thoracic spine, since radicular pain from this area can radiate into the groin. Hip joint movements should be gauged, and particular Trendelenberg tests should be carried out with the patient standing. Any gluteal weakness should be noted. Local tenderness over the adductor region, symphysis pubis or sacrococcygeal area should be assessed by direct palpation. If these assessments are entirely normal an orthopaedic cause for the pelvic pain is unlikely.

Bacteriological Investigation of Genitourinary Infections

E. J. G. Glencross

A microbiologist's interest in pelvic pain in women will inevitably be concerned with infections of the genitourinary tract, and while pelvic inflammatory disease will take centre stage, other infections in this area can also conveniently be considered.

Urinary Tract Infection

Women with attacks of frequent and painful micturition make up a considerable proportion of a general practitioner's workload and generate a large number of specimens for a microbiology department. When infection is confined to the lower urinary tract, frequency and dysuria are the main symptoms, while the addition of loin pain, tenderness in the renal angle and pyrexia indicate that the kidney is also involved. Invasive diagnostic techniques are not indicated in the majority of patients. In pyelonephritis the urine will contain significant numbers of bacteria, whereas in women with infection confined to the lower urinary tract bacteria can be demonstrated in only about half of the cases. The term "urethral syndrome" is sometimes applied to this symptomatic abacteriuria. About 5 % of women have the reverse condition – significant bacteriuria in the absence of symptoms. This does not require treatment in the adult except in pregnancy, when severe pyelonephritis may occur, usually in the second trimester.

It is now accepted that infection, except in neonates, in whom infection may be haematogenous, almost invariably occurs by the ascending route, and is commonly due to aerobic Gram negative bacilli, of which *Escherichia coli* is by far the commonest species. A second major pathogen, *Staphylococcus saprophyticis*, occurs in women of childbearing age. The reason for this is unclear but may be associated with sexual intercourse, which generally facilitates the entry of bacteria from the introitus to the bladder. Here bacterial multiplication is encouraged by the stagnation of urine overnight. An inadequate fluid intake during the day will have the same effect.

The management of women with urinary tract infection will depend on a number of factors and is outlined in Table 2.3.

For patients presenting with a first attack in the sexually active period a short course of antibiotics and advice on frequent and complete micturition may be all that is required. Repeated attacks must be investigated by examination of a carefully collected midstream specimen of urine, followed initially by appropriate antibiotic therapy. For those women with negative cultures and the urethral syndrome further antibiotics are best avoided, as there is some evidence that repeat courses may encourage the colonisation of the urethra and surrounding tissue with resistant lactobacilli. These women may obtain some relief from the alkalinisation of the urine with potassium citrate. Women who have persistent or relapsing bacteriuria, pyuria or haematuria after appropriate therapy and those with associated hypertension should be referred for urological investigation. Other causes of this syndrome may be related to fastidious microorganisms not identified by the usual routine culture of urine. Women may also complain of dysuria when the underlying pathology is a vaginitis or a sexually transmitted disease.

Because of the workload involved, most laboratories use a simple method for the routine examination of urines. This involves a dipstick method for

Table 2.3. Management of women with urinary tract infection

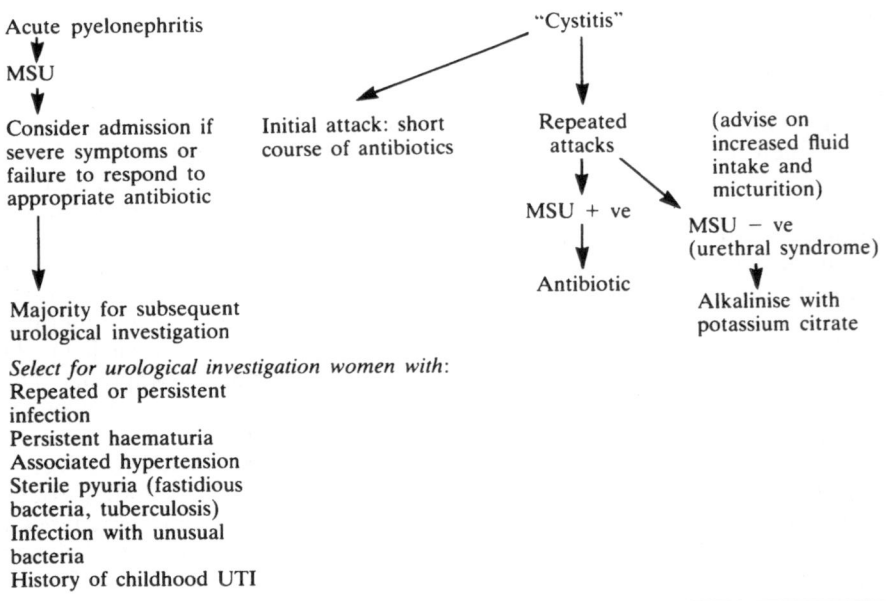

MSU, midstream urine; UTI, urinary tract infection

Table 2.4. Factors which affect interpretation of urine culture

Method of collection	Presence of pyuria
Age of specimen	Pure or mixed culture
Frequency	Type of specimen (MSU/catheter)
Inhibitory substance (antibiotic)	Sex of patient

MSU, midstream urine.

the presence of protein and glucose, the microscopy of an uncentrifuged specimen for pyuria and a semiquantitative method of urine culture. This involves a known volume of urine being cultured overnight on a solid medium, the resultant growth being assessed as significant or otherwise. Infected and contaminated urine specimens from females without urinary symptoms can be distinguished by bacterial count. In a pure culture a count of more than 10^5/ml indicates a significant bacterial infection of the urinary tract; counts below 10^3/ml indicate contamination, and intermediate values justify repeat examination. This arithmetical approach is used by many laboratories as an aid to the interpretation of culture results from women with symptoms. However, since the number of bacteria that can be cultured from urine is affected by a variety of factors (Table 2.4) such interpretation must be done with caution.

In an ideal world a midstream specimen of urine collected after careful vulval toilet would arrive at the laboratory and be examined within 2 hours. Specimens from domiciliary and hospital practice often fail to meet this high ideal, but bacterial multiplication can be delayed by using a dip-culture technique in the surgery or by transferring the specimen to a bacteriostatic transport medium such as boric acid.

A high fluid intake is encouraged to improve the flushing action of micturition and, where relevant, micturition is encouraged after sexual intercourse. For women with infection confined to the lower urinary tract a 2–3 day course of antibiotics will help tip the balance in favour of the normal clearance mechanisms. Selection of an antibiotic will depend on local sensitivity patterns, side-effects and cost. A typical series of over 2000 significant isolates from domiciliary practice has shown sensitivities to the following antibiotics: ampicillin 62.1 %, sulphonamide 62.7 %, trimethoprim 80.5 % and cephradine 82.9 %. Taking into account the higher cost of cephradine, an initial first choice before sensitivity results are available in the individual case would be trimethoprim. Failure to respond to a short course of an appropriate antibiotic may indicate the need for more extensive urological investigation.

In acute pyelonephritis a longer course of antibiotics is indicated, and as these may have to be given parenterally admission to hospital is usually required. In patients with recurring symptoms and persistent bacteriuria with radiological abnormalities, long-term antibiotic suppression may be required. Trimethoprim and nitrofurantoin given last thing at night have been successfully used. It is usual to assess such therapy every 6 months with frequent urine examinations on a serial basis or at recurrence of symptoms.

Vaginal Discharge

Under this heading is discussed the abnormal discharge associated with inflammation of the vaginal walls. Infection of the cervix and urethra, which may also cause discharge, is considered under the heading of Sexually Transmitted Diseases.

Candida albicans

Small numbers of yeast cells are sometimes found in the vaginal flora of normal women. Increase in numbers, often associated with a precipitating cause such as diabetes, pregnancy or use of antibiotics, results in a white thick irritating discharge. Diagnosis can be confirmed by collecting the discharge on a charcoal-coated swab and sending this to the laboratory in a transport medium such as Stuart's medium. Here microscopy or the more sensitive culture methods will reveal the presence of candida species.

Treatment is by the insertion of nystatin vaginal pessaries for at least 14 days or one of the imidazole drugs which, though expensive, often cure after one application.

Trichomonas vaginalis

This is a flagellated protozoan, and infection causes a thin frothy offensive discharge. Transmission is mainly by sexual intercourse. The diagnosis can be confirmed by sending a swab collected as for candida infections. Microscopy will reveal the characteristic motility of the protozoon, and this is retained for at least 24 hours in a suitable transport medium. Some laboratories also apply a culture technique, which is slightly more sensitive than microscopy alone.

Treatment is by metronidazole, 200 mg every 8 hours for 7 days, with simultaneous treatment of the male partner.

Non-specific Vaginitis

There is increasing evidence that large numbers of anaerobes in association with *Gardnerella vaginalis* can be responsible for nonspecific vaginal discharge. While these can be present in normal women, the complete syndrome is an association of a thin malodorous discharge, "clue" cells and a vaginal pH above 4.5. These clue cells are epithelial cells with an attached covering of gardnerella and are easily visible by microscopical examination of wet preparations.

A swab collected as for candida or trichomonas infection is suitable for the isolation of *G. vaginalis*. Metronidazole 400 mg twice daily for 7 days is an effective therapy and is believed to act mainly on the associated anaerobes. Other bacteria are frequently isolated from vaginal sections and reflect colonisation or contamination rather than infection. An exception to this is infection with *Streptococcus pyogenes*, which sometimes causes post-menopausal vaginitis.

Important Sexually Transmitted Diseases

Interest in the sexually transmitted diseases has been rekindled in the last few years by the development of penicillinase producing gonococci, genital herpes and the progress of acquired immune deficiency syndrome (AIDS). Fear of genital herpes and, more particularly, AIDS has led to some modification of sexual behaviour. This could have a permanent effect on reducing the incidence of sexually acquired disease.

Gonococcal Infection

Neisseria gonorrhoeae is very susceptible to drying, and this susceptibility both limits the method of spread to contact with a fresh infected discharge and makes laboratory detection difficult. In the adult female of childbearing age infection is initially limited to the endocervix and urethra. The infection may be associated with a purulent discharge with frequency and dysuria, but a high percentage of infected women are symptomless. Other mucous membranes such as the throat and rectum are also susceptible, and here again the infection may be occult.

Local spread may cause acute barthinolitis, but it is an ascending infection with acute salpingitis which is the most important complication. This will be considered later under the heading of Pelvic Inflammatory Disease.

The laboratory confirmation of gonorrhoea is made on swabs from the cervix and urethra and submitted in a suitable bacterial transport medium. Kits issued for the investigation of trichomoniasis or candidiasis are suitable for this, but the swabs must be collected from the endocervix and urethra. While the gonococcus is sometimes isolated from high vaginal swabs, this is not a sensitive enough method when the suspicion index is high.

Culture techniques involve the use of a highly selective medium, and subsequent isolates are identified by biochemical and serological means. Direct examination with Gram staining of exudates is not sufficiently sensitive and specific to replace culture techniques. While the initial diagnosis can be made in domiciliary practice, referral to a specialist clinic is essential to allow contact tracing to limit spread of the disease.

Treatment of uncomplicated gonorrhoea is usually by single-dose ampicillin 3 g orally or procaine penicillin 2.4 megaunits intramuscularly (IM), each given with 2 g oral probenecid. In areas where penicillin resistance is high, spectinomycin 2 g IM or cefotaxime 1 g IM are suitable alternatives. Cultures must be repeated 1–2 weeks after therapy as a test for cure.

Chlamydial Infection

Chlamydia were once thought to be viruses but are now regarded as bacteria which lack the ability to multiply extracellularly. Certain serotypes of *Chlamydia trachomatis* (D–K) primarily infect the genital tract and in men cause approximately half the cases of non-gonococcal urethritis and are now a more common cause of urethritis than the gonococcus.

In women chlamydia can be isolated from the cervix and urethra in up to 25% of those attending clinics for sexually transmitted diseases, but symptoms are much less dramatic than in men. Nevertheless, there is evidence that some cases of hypertrophic cervicitis and the urethral syndrome may be due to infection and that *C. trachomatis* is the cause of a substantial proportion of cases of acute salpingitis. Neonatal inclusion conjunctivitis follows infection at birth. Chlamydial infection may be detected by serological methods or by detection of the agent within cells. All chlamydia have a common group antigen, and a complement fixation test will also demonstrate antibodies following infection with *C. psittaci* and the serotypes of *C. trachomatis* causing lymphogranuloma venereum. It is this non-specific nature of the response in the complement fixation test and the persistence of antibodies in the absence of current infection which limit the diagnostic value of this test unless a rise in titre can be demonstrated. A more specific and sensitive serological test depending on microimmunofluorescence is not generally available.

Direct microscopy of exudate for chlamydial intracellular inclusions is too insensitive for routine use, but isolation of the agent in tissue culture is both sensitive and specific. Laboratories with virology expertise and experienced in tissue culture techniques may offer this service on swabs of exudate collected in chlamydial transport medium. Expense and the labour intensive nature of the investigation limit the application of this service.

Commercial enzyme immunoassay kits which demonstrate chlamydial antigen in infected discharges are now available to most laboratories. However, this method is not as specific or as sensitive as culture techniques in the most experienced hands. In the absence of laboratory confirmation the status of the sexual partner may be the most valuable indicator to the diagnosis of infection in the female.

Treatment of uncomplicated infection of the cervix and urethra depends on the use of tetracycline. Doxycycline 200 mg orally daily for 7–14 days is often prescribed. Erythromycin 500 mg orally 4 times daily is substituted in pregnancy.

Mycoplasma Infections

Mycoplasmas can be looked upon as bacteria which do not possess a cell wall. Like bacteria they can multiply on a suitable cell free medium. In human beings at least 11 species can be identified, including *Mycoplasma pneumoniae*, one cause of atypical pneumonia, and *M. hominis* and *Ureaplasma urealyticans*. The last two species are capable of colonising the genital tract and are frequently isolated in the absence of disease in the sexually promiscuous. There is some evidence that *M. hominis* is occasionally related to pelvic inflammatory disease and post-partum fever, and *U. urealyticans* is isolated from some cases of non-gonococcal urethritis in men. In routine laboratory practice the investigation of genital mycoplasmas is rarely called for, and when treatment is required the organism will respond to tetracycline and erythromycin.

Uncommon Sexually Transmitted Bacterial Infections

Other bacterial infections causing ulceration of the genital tract include syphilis, the mainly tropical disease chancroid (*Haemophilus ducreyi*), granuloma inguinale (*Calymmatobacterium granulomatis*) and lymphogranuloma venereum (*Chlamydia trachomatis* serotypes I, II and III). All require treatment by a specialist in sexually transmitted diseases.

Genital Herpes

This extremely common and unpleasant virus infection is due to the herpes simplex virus (HSV). Two strains of this virus exist, type 2 causing most genital infections. A characteristic of the herpes group of viruses is their ability to establish a persistent latent infection in the host. Approximately half of all patients have repeated attacks.

The primary infection usually starts some 7 days after the initial sexual contact, with localised burning and pain in the back and buttocks. Groups of small papules develop on the mucosal surface of the labia minora and may spread to the labia majora and surrounding skin. Vesicles develop within 1–2 days and soon rupture, leaving shallow and painful ulcers which gradually heal over the next 2 weeks. Severe attacks are frequently associated with constitutional symptoms of malaise and pyrexia. Dysuria can be a prominent and distressing symptom. Lesions may also develop on the cervix, and even in their absence virus may be shed from this site. Perianal lesions can cause severe pain on defaecation, as can the associated proctitis.

Recurrent attacks are usually not so severe as the primary infection and often the whole development and healing is accelerated. The trigger mechanism for recurrence may be menstruation, sunlight, stress or fever, and it is suggested that these factors interfere with the local defence mechanisms, allowing any virus present to replicate and cause the mucocutaneous lesions.

Diagnosis is usually made on clinical grounds, but when laboratory confirmation is required a swab of vesicle fluid collected into virus transport medium allows the isolation of HSV in tissue culture. This will take up to a week. Electron microscopy and the more specific method of direct immunofluorescence of clinical material using specific antiviral serum will allow confirmation within a couple of hours.

A primary attack can be diagnosed serologically from the rise in antibody levels. In recurrent herpes, however, the rise in titre is minimal.

Treatment of genital herpes is with acyclovir, which inhibits the replication of the virus and so must be used as early as possible either in topical or systemic form. Cream containing 5% acyclovir applied four or five times daily assists healing and reduces viral shedding. If the lesions are extensive or cervical, then oral therapy with 200 mg given five times daily for 5 days is indicated. Very severe infection, which necessitates admission to hospital, can be treated intravenously, but no initial regimen appears to affect the frequency of recurrence. Very frequent and severe recurrences can be suppressed with oral acyclovir given in slightly reduced dosage over extended periods, with interruptions every 6 months or so for reassessment. There appear to be no side-effects.

While infection with hepatitis B and human immunodeficiency viruses are of enormous clinical importance as sexually transmitted diseases, they are not directly related to pelvic pain. Genital warts caused by papillomavirus, although extremely common, also fall into this category.

Pelvic Inflammatory Disease

Secondary pelvic infection may follow surgery, septic abortion or pregnancy due to the entry of endogenous bacteria into the damaged pelvic tissues. This section, however, will concentrate on primary acute salpingitis (Table 2.5).

There is increasing evidence that primary acute salpingitis in younger women generally follows infection of the cervix with *Neisseria gonorrhoeae, Chlamydia trachomatis* or more uncommonly *Mycoplasma hominis*. The mechanism by which infection ascends from the cervix to the endosalpinx is unknown, but it has been suggested that gonococci may ascend attached to spermatozoa.

While infection at the time of sampling from the endosalpinx may be polymicrobial, it is not known whether this usually follows an initiating venereal infection or whether bacteria colonising the normal vagina may be the primary pathogens. The consequences of salpingitis, apart from spread of infection into the peritoneal cavity, including perihepatitis, may eventually result in a partial or complete occlusion of the Fallopian tubes, with an increased likelihood of ectopic pregnancy or infertility. This may follow a single acute attack, especially if therapy is delayed or ineffective. It is particularly likely to follow chlamydial salpingitis, which may present as an apparently benign infection.

One of the factors associated with an increase in pelvic inflammatory disease is the fitting of an intrauterine contraceptive device (IUCD). In older women, particularly, infection may be due to endogenous bacteria such as coliforms and anaerobes.

Infection associated with an IUCD seems to be less likely if the device contains copper, which is probably bactericidal. Bacterial colonisation of the uterine cavity is believed to be facilitated by the tail of the IUCD, which interferes with the normal plug of cervical mucus. There is also evidence

Table 2.5. Pelvic inflammatory disease

Older age group	Younger age group
Causes	
Tissue damage	Primary acute salpingitis
Surgery	IUCD
Pregnancy	
Abortion	
IUCD	
Organisms	
Pyogenic endogenous bacteria	Sexually transmitted *Chlamydia trachomatis*, *Neisseria gonorrhoeae* + secondary invaders
Investigations	
Blood culture	Cervical swab
Cervical swab	Laparoscopy specimens
Treatment	
Beta-lactam antibiotic	Tetracycline
Aminoglycosides	Metronidazole
Metronidazole	Additional for gonorrhoea

IUCD, intrauterine contraceptive device.

that colonisation of the cervix with actinomyces-like organisms may occur with plastic devices. These microorganisms are seen in cervical smears and are possibly associated with pain and purulent discharge. Removal of the IUCD and replacement with a copper device usually results in a negative smear without the need for antibiotic therapy.

Laparoscopy is being increasingly used to support a clinical diagnosis of acute salpingitis based on bilateral lower abdominal pain and tenderness. The procedure also allows the collection of specimens for microbiology. It is generally considered that gonorrhoeal associated infection is the most florid and that patients are more likely to consult after a short period of abdominal pain and be referred for hospital advice.

The demonstration of *C. trachomatis* or *N. gonorrhoeae* in a cervical discharge is evidence but not absolute proof of the aetiology of a pelvic inflammatory infection. This is even more so when cervical isolates are confined to anaerobes or coliform bacteria, which are frequently found in the absence of pelvic disease. Specimens obtained at laparoscopy may be more significant, especially if collected early in the infection, but pus from the Fallopian tubes is not usually available to the microbiologist. Isolation of the gonococcus from cervix, urethra or Fallopian tube is more likely during the first infection than subsequently, but failure to isolate this organism or chlamydia in any relevant specimen is not unusual.

Because of the polymicrobial nature of pelvic inflammatory disease and the need for early therapy before the results of microbiology are available, it is customary to use a combination of antibiotics, to cover as many options as possible. Tetracycline 500 mg four times daily and metronidazole 400 mg three times daily given orally for 10–14 days should be effective against

C. trachomatis, *M. hominis*, anaerobes and most strains of *N. gonorrhoeae*. Should tetracycline resistance be a problem with local strains of gonococci then ampicillin 3 g with pobenecid 2 g orally followed by 0.5 g of both 6-hourly for 10 days, or spectinomycin 2 g IM twice a day for 10 days may be added to the regimen. Contact tracing and subsequent treatment of sexual partners completes the cure.

Treatment of pelvic infection following abortion, surgery or pregnancy is more likely to be directly guided by the microbiology of the cervical discharge and is usually a combination of a beta-lactam antibiotic or aminoglycoside plus metronidazole.

Chronic Pelvic Infection

Progression to chronic pelvic infection associated with chronic pelvic pain, dyspareunia and general ill-health can be greatly reduced by effective antibiotic therapy given during the acute stage of infection. At operation the contents of the diseased Fallopian tubes are usually sterile.

Specific chronic infections are the rare actinomycosis (usually an extension from intestinal disease) and tuberculosis. The latter is usually secondary to infection elsewhere and is often demonstrated following diagnostic curettage for menorrhagia or infertility. If amenorrhoea is present then the histology becomes more typical of tuberculosis. Tubercle bacilli may be isolated from curettings sent to the laboratory dry in a sterile container.

Treatment with triple antituberculous therapy is best supervised by a physician with special experience, but surgery may eventually prove necessary, especially in the presence of a pelvic mass.

Summary of Common Diagnostic Specimens (Table 2.6)

The exact nature of the materials and methods used will depend on the local laboratory, but in general swabs should be submitted in the appropriate transport medium with minimum delay. If delay is unavoidable refrigeration is permissible for up to 24 hours. Such refrigeration also applies to urine samples.

Clinical information is essential for assessing the relevance of pyogenic bacteria isolated from vaginal specimens. Although important in secondary pelvic sepsis, they frequently represent a temporary vaginal colonisation rather than true infection.

Diagnostic Imaging

A. Jones

The radiologist has a wide range of modalities with which to work, but the meaningful choice of a particular radiological technique and its interpretation depends on good clinical information.

Table 2.6. Diagnostic specimens: pelvic inflammatory disease

Site	Transport medium			Isolation/ identification
	Bacterial	Chlamydial	Virus	
High vaginal	✓			*Candida albicans* *Trichomonas vaginalis* *Gardnerella vaginalis* Pyogenic bacteria, including anaerobes
Cervical os	✓			*Neisseria gonorrhoeae*
		✓		*Chlamydia trachomatis*
			✓[a]	Herpes simplex virus
Urethral os	✓			*N. gonorrhoeae*

[a] Also from vesicles in other sites.

In the majority of patients with pelvic pain a detailed clinical history and examination will indicate whether the disease is gynaecological, urinary, intestinal or musculoskeletal in origin, and the discussion of radiological investigation in this chapter is based on systematic investigation.

Gynaecological Disease

In the investigation of gynaecological disease plain film radiography is only rarely helpful. Sonography, when interpreted with the full clinical picture, can be valuable. In certain circumstances, such as pelvic abscess and staging of malignancy, computed tomography can be helpful.

The question of when to perform pelvic sonography is difficult to answer. Certainly when clinical examination indicates a definite or suspected gynaecological mass then pelvic sonography is recommended. In patients with a history suggesting a gynaecological problem but in whom clinical examination is normal the expected return from pelvic sonography is variable.

The usual sonographic approach to the pelvis is transabdominal, a distended urinary bladder being used as an acoustic window. The distended bladder displaces gas-containing bowel upwards and also straightens the normally anteverted uterus (Fig. 2.1) so that it can be viewed along its length. The more recently introduced vaginal transducers (probes), being of higher frequency and getting closer to the uterus and adnexa, give more detail and do not require a distended bladder. Endovaginal scanning will not be suitable for all patients, and the reduced penetration of high-frequency ultrasound will limit its use to smaller gynaecological masses. Even so, more detailed sonographic images should improve diagnostic accuracy and will be helpful for use in obese patients, where both clinical assessment and transabdominal sonography are difficult.

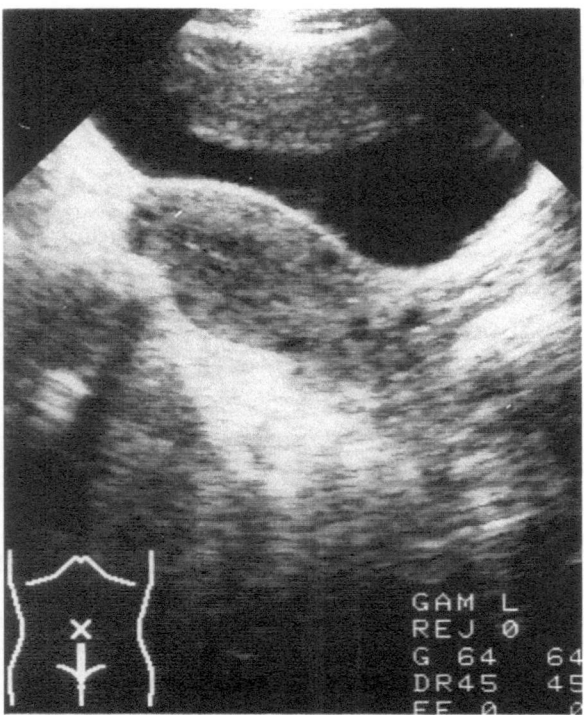

Fig. 2.1. Ultrasonograph showing normally anteverted uterus and hypoechoic areas of adenomyosis.

The purpose of pelvic ultrasonography is to demonstrate any deviation from the norm in the uterus or adnexa and to detect the presence of any abnormal structure or abnormal fluid collection in the pelvic cavity. It is usually possible to determine the site of a pelvic mass (e.g., uterine or ovarian) but occasionally finding a plane of cleavage between a paraovarian or parauterine mass can be difficult. Furthermore considerable diagnostic difficulty can be encountered in widespread pelvic disease, when the outlines of the uterus and adnexa are ill defined.

In the majority of cases sonography can specify disease at a particular site, but a definitive or histological diagnosis cannot be expected. However, if sonographic features are interpreted with the full clinical picture, then a good presumptive diagnosis is attained.

Uterus

Sonography can detect change in size, shape or outline of the uterus and can assess alteration in the normally uniform echo pattern of the myometrium. Sonographic evaluation of the endometrium is more difficult because of variation of endometrial echoes related to the menstrual cycle, hormonal therapy, age, etc. However, displacement of the endometrium by a myometrial mass is more readily demonstrated, and focal areas of disease in the endometrium can be demonstrated with high-resolution sonography.

Sonographic evaluation of the retroverted uterus is difficult, and a normal retroverted uterus can appear "bulky".

Excluding gestational problems, the abnormal uterus can be assessed as follows:

1. Enlargement can be due to neoplasm (benign/malignant), adenomyosis, or fluid collection in the uterine cavity (haematometra/hydrometra/pyometra).
2. Shape can be altered by neoplasm or congenital abnormality.
3. Outline can be lobulated as a result of neoplasm or surgical procedure and can become ill defined through pelvic inflammatory disease or endometriosis.
4. Myometrial echo pattern can be altered by adenomyosis (Fig. 2.1), neoplasm or degenerative change or necrosis in a neoplasm.
5. Endometrial echo pattern varies with the stage of menstruation and can show increased echo pattern resulting from endometrial hyperplasia/polyps, endometritis and retained products of conception.

In essence, uterine structural changes can be demonstrated by sonography, but definitive diagnosis cannot confidently be provided. Even when a uterine mass shows rapid increase in size on sequential scans it is not possible to be sure whether this is due to degenerative change or a transition from a benign to a malignant condition.

Adnexa

In women of reproductive age normal ovaries are usually oval, measure 3–4 cm in their longest diameter and contain a few follicles. Typically, polycystic ovaries are enlarged and rounded and have multiple follicles of varying size. Ovarian masses can be divided into three main sonographic groups:

1. Cystic masses include functional cysts, cystadenoma, cystic teratoma, ovarian abscess and endometrioma.
2. Mixed cystic/solid masses include cystadenoma/cystadenocarcinoma, dermoid, granulosa cell tumour and implanted ectopic.
3. Solid masses are rare but include adenocarcinoma, benign/malignant teratoma, metastases to the ovary and fibroma.

Radiology will clearly show the "diagnostic" tooth of a dermoid (Fig. 2.2). Serial scanning can be helpful in assessing cyclical regression in functional ovarian cysts or response of an abscess treated with antibiotics, but generally no definite diagnosis can be expected from sonography.

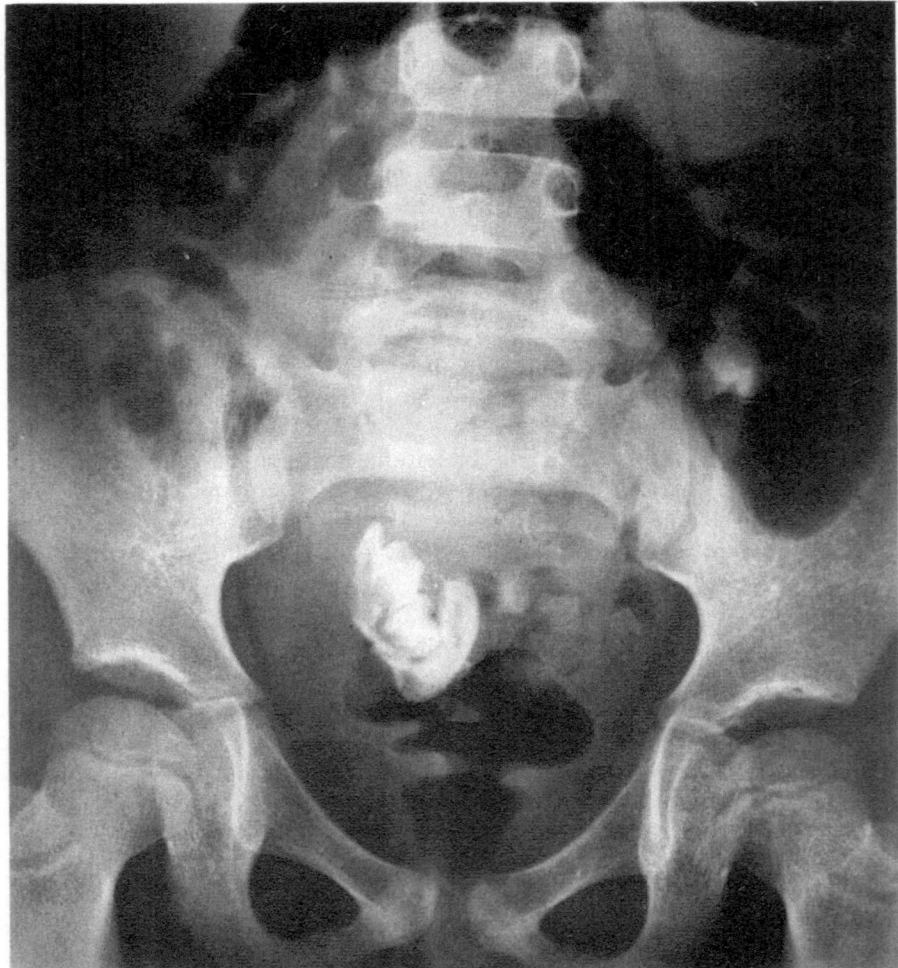

Fig. 2.2. Radiological appearance of teeth in an ovarian dermoid.

Pelvic Inflammatory Disease

Sonographic features of pelvic inflammatory disease vary depending on the stage of the disease and the areas involved. In acute pelvic inflammatory disease sonography may be normal or may demonstrate ill-defined outlines of pelvic organs, excess fluid in the pouch of Douglas or a mixed cystic/ solid adnexal mass. Although tubo-ovarian abscess is often adnexal in position as opposed to a dependent pelvic abscess (due to remote abdominal disease) which occupies the pouch of Douglas even this differentiation cannot be relied upon, as adnexal structures not uncommonly lie in the pouch of Douglas.

With chronic pelvic inflammatory disease the sonographic features can become even more complicated, with further ill-definition of anatomical outlines and an extremely complicated picture in the presence of gut adhesions, hydrosalpinx etc.

Occasionally an abscess can be diagnosed when gas bubbles are detected in a mass, but generally pelvic inflammatory disease can mimic endometriosis, ovarian cyst rupture, ectopic gestation and the complications of remote abdominal disease causing pelvic abscess or adhesions.

Ectopic Pregnancy

About 1% of all pregnancies are ectopic. The majority of ectopic implantations are tubal, mainly isthmic or ampullary, and at the time of diagnosis most have undergone tubal rupture.

In suspected ectopic gestation, pelvic sonography is usually performed, and ideally the result of a sensitive pregnancy test should be available to the sonologist.

Sonography in early normal pregnancy shows a little uterine enlargement and an intrauterine gestation sac with surrounding decidual reaction. Later a small foetal pole within the sac will be discernible. Foetal viability can usually be demonstrated by 8 weeks' gestation and possibly earlier (especially with endovaginal sonography). However, many patients with possible ectopic pregnancy present before foetal viability is demonstrable and sometimes at a stage where even demonstration of a definite foetal pole can be difficult.

In suspected ectopic pregnancy the most useful sonographic result is the demonstration of a normal intrauterine gestational sac containing a viable foetus, and in such a situation the likelihood of a twin ectopic is in the order of 1 : 30 000 (although some recent publications suggest 1 : 10 000).

When ectopic implantation has occurred it is uncommon to be able to demonstrate a definite extrauterine gestation sac and rare to be able to demonstrate a viable extrauterine foetus.

An adnexal mass due to other disease can mimic an ectopic implantation and vice versa. Furthermore, in ectopic pregnancy there can be a pseudogestational sac in the uterine cavity with a surrounding single layer of decidual reaction, but in true uterine implantation the decidual reaction may be shown to be a double layer representing the decidua vera and capsularis.

In suspected ectopic pregnancy clinical action depends on the results of pregnancy test, sonography and the patient's clinical condition. If there is doubt, laparoscopy is indicated.

Urinary Tract Disease

When clinical assessment indicates disease of the lower urinary tract, then with few exceptions the initial radiological investigation should be intravenous

Fig. 2.3a   Pelvic calculus.

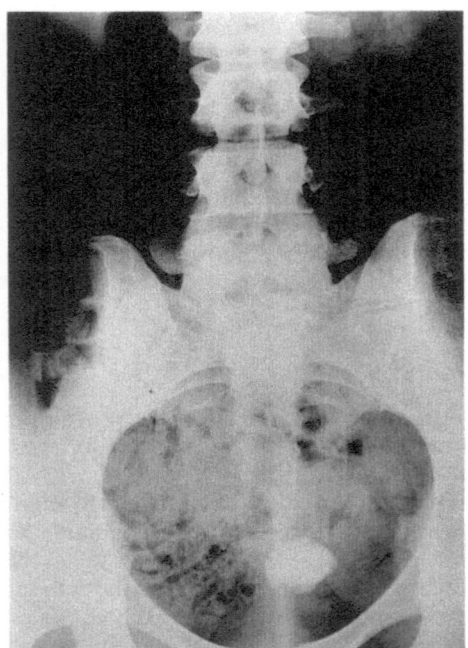

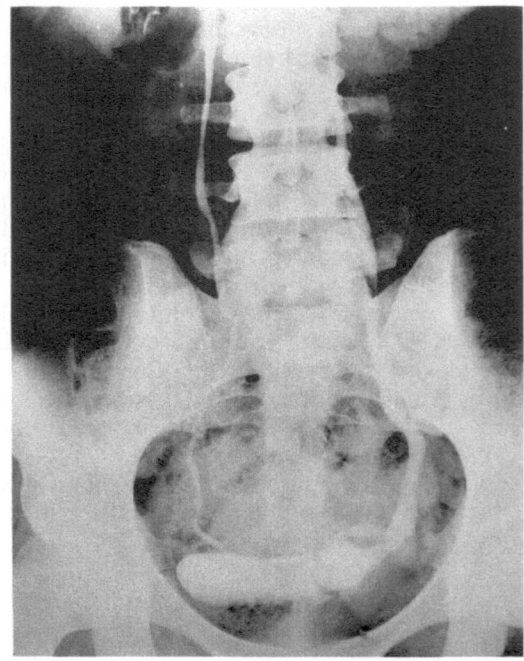

Fig. 2.3b   TVU showing calculus in ureterocele.

urography (IVU). Some exceptions to this are bladder dysfunction, cystitis in young women, and suspected enterovesical fistula. These are discussed below.

Urinary Tract Infection

In young women with recurrent urinary tract infection intravenous urography is not routinely recommended. However, IVU is recommended in recurrent urinary tract infection in older women and in young women with additional features such as haematuria, severe diabetes mellitus or a past history of childhood urinary infections, calculus disease or genitourinary surgery.

Primary infection of the upper urinary tract is not considered here.

Cystitis

IVU can show changes resulting from chronic cystitis, but further pathological investigation or cystoscopy is usually necessary for a definitive diagnosis.

In bacterial cystitis the bladder usually appears normal on IVU. Rarely there may be mucosal oedema, but bladder wall contracture due to fibrosis is extremely rare.

Emphysematous cystitis is a rare condition usually occurring in patients with severe diabetes who have a bladder outflow problem. The causative organism is usually *Escherichia coli*, and although plain radiographs will often demonstrate the vesical intramural and intraluminal gas, the overall extent of the infection is best demonstrated by IVU.

Both tuberculosis and schistosomiasis of the bladder can show irregular bladder mucosa (even mimicking neoplasia) and in later stages of the disease bladder contracture. In schistosomiasis bladder wall calcification is a diagnostic feature.

Chemical cystitis can cause bladder contracture, but cyclophosphamide cystitis is a haemorrhagic cystitis with intraluminal blood clots and shows on IVU with mucosal swelling and luminal filling defects.

The bladder is extremely resistant to radiation exposure, and usually there are no changes on IVU.

Pelvic Urinary Calculi

The majority of vesical calculi, being radio-opaque, are visible on a plain radiograph and are readily confirmed by IVU. Only occasionally is a radiolucent calculus difficult to differentiate from tumour or blood clot on IVU, but very small calculi can be obscured by contrast medium.

Vesical calculi may be associated with calculi in the upper urinary tract, bladder outflow obstruction or a bladder diverticulum, and a pelvic urinary calculus can originate in a congenital anomaly such as a ureterocele (Fig. 2.3). IVU will demonstrate these associations.

Calculi may be the result of metabolic disorders such as hyperparathyroidism, and there may be clues to indicate such a diagnosis on the control films of the IVU.

Vesical Tumour

The reported sensitivity in the detection of bladder tumours by IVU is variable but with optimum technique sensitivity is probably in the order of 60%–70%. In the context of chronic pelvic pain a bladder tumour would have to be complicated by impairment of ureteric drainage or bladder drainage or by extra vesical tumour extension. Therefore, in patients with a malignant vesical neoplasm and pelvic pain the prognosis is likely to be poor. With IVU it is rarely possible to differentiate a benign from a malignant tumour, a cystogram is also unhelpful in this respect and cystoscopy is essential in the assessment of any bladder mass.

Fistulae to the Urinary Tract in the Pelvis

Enterovesical fistula presents with pneumaturia and/or faecaluria. In such patients the investigation of choice is a computed tomographic (CT) scan of the pelvis without prior bladder instrumentation. If this course is chosen then the CT scan is sensitive in confirming the presence of a fistula by demonstrating gas within the bladder lumen and furthermore will frequently indicate whether large or small bowel is involved. Thereafter a more selective course of investigation is possible to determine the site and the nature of the associated gut disease. Without a CT scan such patients are likely to undergo a series of investigations such as IVU, cystography, micturating cystography, multiple barium studies and cystoscopy, all of which have a low sensitivity in demonstrating enterovesical fistula.

Enteroureteric fistula is rare and usually the result of Crohn's disease. It can present in the same way as enterovesical fistula, and therefore the manner of investigation as indicated above should be followed.

Urinary fistula to the vagina is usually readily demonstrated by IVU, but cystography may give additional information.

Ureteric Disease

Primary disease of the ureter usually presents with upper urinary tract symptoms and is beyond the scope of this text. The ureter may become diseased secondarily to pelvic disorders, and the clinical picture is then more complicated. The pelvic ureter may be compromised as a result of pelvic tumour or inflammatory process or by surgical trauma.

Intravenous urography will adequately demonstrate many of the above complications, but when ureteric obstruction is such that there is poor opacification or non-opacification of the pelvicalyceal system and ureter then retrograde/antegrade pyelography may be necessary to determine the site and extent of ureteric involvement. On occasion nephrostomy drainage may be necessary. Such cases should be discussed with a radiologist.

Pelvic urinary tract disease can of course cause secondary changes in the upper urinary tracts as a result either of ureteric reflux or of impairment of ureteric drainage. In such situations, micturating cystography or scintigraphy for renal function and ureteric reflux may be necessary.

Congenital Anomalies of the Urinary Tract

Ureterocele, duplication of the urinary tract, ectopic ureter/ectopic ureterocele, ectopic kidney and congenital bladder diverticulum are usually distinctive on IVU. Occasionally a large bladder diverticulum may cause excessive dilution of contrast medium on IVU, and a cystogram may be needed for clearer visualisation.

Preoperative IVU

In patients with or without pelvic masses and whose urinalysis is normal, it has yet to be proven that preoperative IVU reduces the risk of surgical ureteral injury. Even so, many surgeons feel that preoperative knowledge of ureteric anatomy helps avoid ureteric injury, particularly in cases of ureteric duplication.

Bladder Dysfunction

This is best examined by means of urodynamic studies. Micturating cystography for assessment of stress incontinence is outdated, IVU is not recommended, and if assessment of the upper urinary tract is necessary ultrasonography is recommended.

There is a significant incidence of polycystic ovary syndrome in patients with voiding dysfunction, and abnormal electromyographic activity of the urethral sphincter and ultrasonography of the ovaries is recommended in such patients.

Intestinal Disease

The majority of patients with intestinal disease present with symptoms of a chronic bowel disorder and, depending on the clinical situation, will undergo a small bowel or a large bowel barium examination supplemented where necessary by other investigations such as endoscopy and biopsy. A proportion of patients present with an acute abdominal crisis, and these should be considered separately, because barium studies in some of these patients can be hazardous.

Acute Abdominal Crisis

A supine abdominal radiograph and erect chest radiograph to assess subdiaphragmatic gas and chest disease are recommended. The value of an additional erect abdominal radiograph is uncertain, and such a request depends on local practice.

Plain radiographs can be diagnostic of intestinal obstruction, perforation, ileus, volvulus, toxic megacolon, and other forms of megacolon. Plain films may suggest an abscess, a mass, ascites or colitis. Intramural gas, usually streaky in appearance, is a grave sign of intestinal necrosis and is a surgical emergency. It should not be confused with pneumatosis coli/intestinalis, which shows as more rounded intramural bubbles of gas in patients with obstructive airways disease or gastric or duodenal ulceration. Some patients will require further radiological investigation, and the indications and contraindications are discussed below.

Small Bowel Disease

Small bowel disease is investigated by barium examination, and various techniques are used, some of which require jejunal intubation. The best examination of small bowel is obtained if a request is made not for "barium meal and follow-through" but for the more specific "barium examination of small bowel" (BESB).

Acute small bowel obstruction will be demonstrated by a plain radiograph. BESB rarely provides more information and is not recommended.

In *chronic small bowel obstruction* or when clinical assessment indicates small bowel disease BESB can provide valuable information for both diagnosis and management.

Granulomatous disease such as *Crohn's disease* is readily demonstrated by the presence of stricture and ulceration and is most frequently seen in the region of the terminal ileum, but differentiation from *tuberculosis* and *actinomycosis* can be difficult. Similar changes can also be seen in *gut ischaemia* and in *radiation ileitis*.

Tapered narrowing of small bowel can be seen in the presence of *adhesions* or *herniation* of small bowel. *Meckel's diverticulum* is difficult to demonstrate with barium examination, and Meckel's diverticulum symptomatic as a result of ectopic gastric mucosa is best sought by scintigraphy.

Primary tumours of small bowel, which are rare, are usually malignant and most frequently adenocarcinoma, which infiltrates small bowel causing circumferential narrowing. *Carcinoid* tumour can mimic carcinoma, but *lymphosarcoma* tends to expand the wall of the small bowel. *Malignant tumours* very rarely result in intussusception, but the rarer *benign tumours* such as adenoma or lipoma are often pedunculated and can form the apex of an intussusception. *Serosal* involvement of small bowel by metastatic tumour or endometriosis is usually very difficult to demonstrate with barium studies.

Malabsorption conditions can be demonstrated by means of BESB. Occasionally a specific diagnosis can be made, but usually further investigation, including biopsy, will be necessary for a definitive diagnosis.

Colorectal Disease

When *toxic megacolon* or *severe colitis* is suspected a plain abdominal radiograph is necessary. This will confirm the presence of toxic megacolon and frequently will indicate the extent of colitis. Because of the risk of perforation barium enema is absolutely contraindicated in the presence of toxic megacolon and should be avoided in the presence of severe colitis, although in the latter circumstance a limited single-contrast barium enema without bowel cleansing may give diagnostic information.

Barium enema performed after recent colonic biopsy entails a risk of perforation, the risk increasing with the depth of biopsy. It is generally agreed that barium enema should be delayed for 7 days after biopsy via rigid sigmoidoscope and for a few days following biopsy via a fibreoptic endoscope. In patients where *large bowel obstruction* is suspected but plain film findings are equivocal a single-contrast barium enema without bowel cleansing can provide useful information but this should be discussed with the radiologist.

For other situations where large bowel disease is suspected, a double-contrast barium enema (DCBE) is indicated, but this should be preceded at least by a rectal examination and whenever possible by sigmoidoscopy.

DCBE with adequate bowel cleansing is accurate in detecting disease, but a histological diagnosis is not always possible and there are a few diagnostic difficulties. For example, when there is marked diverticular disease, it can be difficult to differentiate an inflammatory stricture from a malignant stricture, and endoscopic assessment will be necessary. Furthermore, in the presence of multiple diverticulae polyps can be missed.

Colitic changes are readily demonstrated by DCBE, and when proposing a specific diagnosis the radiologist places emphasis on the distribution of colitic change – for example, *ulcerative colitis* extends proximally from the rectum, whereas *Crohn's colitis* is variable in distribution but commonly arises in the ileocaecal area and extends distally.

Detection of mild rectal inflammation can be difficult on barium enema, and sigmoidoscopy is therefore essential. Other relevant information, such as the rectal administration of steroid preparations, should be made known to the radiologist. The diagnosis of *ischaemic colitis*, *radiation colitis*, *tuberculous* and *amoebic colitis* depends on the site of colitic change, the history and the likelihood of such disease, and a specific radiological diagnosis is not always possible. DCBE has a high sensitivity in the detection of *colonic neoplasms*. A typical adenocarcinoma with "apple core" deformity rarely presents diagnostic difficulty, and when there is calcification within such a mass, the diagnosis of the rare mucin-secreting *colloid carcinoma* is indicated. However, *polypoidal masses* vary considerably in size and complexity, and although larger polyps with a broad base are more likely to be malignant, benign and malignant polyps cannot confidently be differentiated, and endoscopic assessment will be necessary in such cases. Large-bowel polyps can give rise to discomfort and occasionally form the apex of an intussusception.

An intrarectal ultrasonographic probe can be useful in the assessment of local spread of rectal carcinoma.

Ileocaecal Disease

The ileocaecal area is a frequent site of intestinal disease. Crohn's disease, tuberculosis, actinomycosis, carcinoid and abscess frequently occur in this area and involve both small and large bowel (Fig. 2.4). Radiological assessment of the ileocaecal area may therefore require a combination of both double-contrast barium enema and barium examination of the small bowel.

Complicated Disease of the Intestinal Tract

Barium studies and plain radiographs may show displacement or indentation of gut, indicating disease or a mass adjacent to the intestinal tract. The barium study may indicate that the primary disease lies in the intestinal system, e.g., diverticular disease with paracolic abscess. On occasion the primary disease lies outside the intestinal tract, and further investigation is necessary to determine its nature. Ultrasonography and computed tomography are valuable in such situations: if abscess is demonstrated percutaneous drainage or aspiration can be considered, and if a solid mass is seen percutaneous biopsy can be arranged.

Intestinal Fistula

Fistulous communication can occur from one part of the intestinal tract to another or from the intestinal tract to another area, such as the urinary system, the genital tract or soft tissues (forming an abscess or cutaneous fistula). A fistula is usually the result of an inflammatory process or a complication of a surgical procedure, but occasionally a malignant tumour is the cause.

Barium examination can confirm the presence of a fistula and indicate the nature of the underlying disease, but inflammation may prevent the flow of contrast medium into a fistulous tract. In suspected rectal communication to a *presacral abscess* or leak from a distal *colonic anastomosis*, it is advisable to request a water-soluble contrast enema, since extravasated barium can interfere with future contrast examinations and occasionally may initiate a foreign-body reaction.

Enterovesical fistulae are discussed in the section on the urinary tract.

Irritable Bowel Syndrome

There is clinical disagreement as to the incidence of irritable bowel syndrome and the manner in which such a diagnosis is made, i.e., history alone or by excluding other pathology.

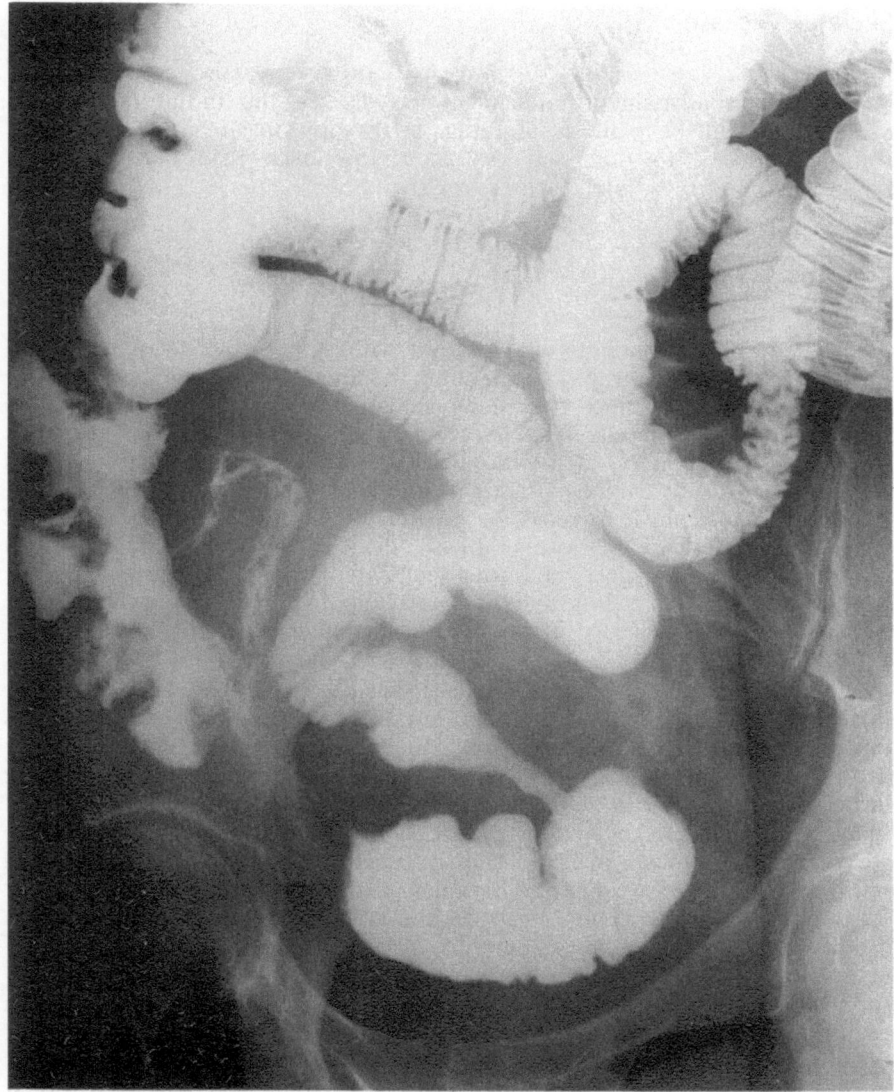

Fig. 2.4. Crohn's disease. Small-bowel barium enema showing stricture of the terminal ileum and contracture of the caecum.

Colonic spasm during barium enema examination is not unusual, and many radiologists routinely use an intravenous hypotonic agent to combat such spasm. Barium enema should be considered a means to detect structural changes and not a means to diagnose colonic spasm.

Skeletal Disease

When clinical assessment indicates bone disease the initial radiological examination will be plain radiography of the appropriate area. There are some exceptions to this, such as acute low back pain and suspected metastases, and these are discussed below.

Low Back Pain

In the majority of patients who present with a first episode of acute low back pain, plain radiography of the lumbar spine is not recommended, since such pain is usually due to conditions which cannot be diagnosed with plain radiographs and pain correlates poorly with any demonstrated degenerative disease. The majority of such patients will, with rest, analgesia and reassurance, return to normal activity in a short period of time. However, if pain is increasing in severity or protracted or if there are neurological signs, then radiological investigation is indicated, particularly if the results of laboratory tests suggest conditions such as bone tumour or infection. The purpose of plain-film radiography is not to demonstrate degenerative disease but to assess the presence of other disorders that can mimic degenerative or discogenic disease.

When pain and neurological signs suggest discogenic disease in the lower lumbar spine then computed tomography (CT) is recommended, since it is more accurate than radiculography in the assessment of lateral disc protrusion. Spinal stenosis is readily demonstrated by CT. However, if it is difficult to determine a neurological level or if spinal tumour is suspected then myelography is indicated (magnetic resonance imaging, if available, would be preferable). In some centres facetography and discography are performed in the assessment of backache and discogenic disease.

Spondylolysthesis, secondary to degenerative change or spondylolysis, is usually diagnosed on plain radiographs, although oblique radiographic views or tomography may be necessary to differentiate degenerative from spondylolytic spondylolysthesis. Occasionally the diagnosis of spondylolysis requires other techniques, such as bone scintigraphy or CT, and differential diagnosis of the rare pedicle tumour must be kept in mind.

Development anomalies of the lumbosacral spine, such as transitional vertebra and rotated or asymmetrical facets, can cause low-back pain.

True spina bifida rarely presents diagnostic difficulty, but the radiological diagnosis of "spina bifida occulta" should be interpreted with great caution. In around one-fifth of the adult population a bony defect is evident in the posterior arch of vertebrae in the lumbosacral area and, in the absence of other clinical factors (neurological/urological), such a defect should be regarded as a common developmental anomaly for which no clinical action is necessary.

Focal Bone Pain

When pain is localised to a particular bony area or a particular joint, plain-film radiography frequently provides the diagnosis and no further radiological examination is needed. This is usually true with degenerative or inflammatory joint disease, and in such cases follow-up radiography to assess the progress of disease is usually unhelpful and is not recommended unless surgical intervention is being considered.

Paget's disease is usually obvious on plain films, but occasionally bone scintigraphy will be necessary to help differentiate it from sclerotic metastases.

Although the degree of bone loss in osteoporosis cannot be accurately assessed by means of plain radiographs, secondary changes such as vertebral body collapse are obvious, and if the vertebral pedicles are intact the likelihood of metastatic disease is remote. However, in such patients the possibility of myeloma should be considered.

Sacroiliitis and ankylosing spondylitis are usually evident on plain films, and only rarely is bone scintigraphy helpful.

Primary bone tumour, benign or malignant, is usually readily demonstrated by plain radiographs, and a presumptive diagnosis based on radiographic appearance and clinical features can be made, but definitive diagnosis frequently requires further investigation, such as bone scintigraphy, magnetic resonance imaging (if available) and biopsy. Early skeletal metastases may not be evident on plain films, and when bone metastases are likely the best approach is bone scintigraphy followed by radiography of suspicious areas.

Infection of bone and joints can be diagnosed on plain films, but the intention of modern practice is to diagnose and treat infection before bone change or cartilage loss is evident on plain films. Diagnosis is therefore usually bacteriological following aspiration of synovial fluid or periostial biopsy, but in doubtful cases bone scintigraphy, showing increased activity in the presence of normal radiographs and clinical suspicion of infection, can focus clinical attention. When infection is suspected around a hip prosthesis, an isotope scan (gallium) can be valuable.

The sacrum can be considerably affected by disease and yet appear normal on plain films. When, rarely, pain indicates focal bone disease in the sacrum and further radiological investigation becomes necessary, bone scintigraphy can be difficult to interpret because of isotope activity in the urinary bladder, and computed tomography may give more information.

Radiological examination for the investigation of coccygeal pain is almost always unhelpful and is not recommended.

Computed Tomography in Pelvic Disease

CT is useful in the staging of pelvic malignant disease and in assessing the response to therapy. It can also be helpful in assessing recurrent rectal carcinoma after resection.

CT is also useful in the detection and assessment of pelvic abscess, and CT guided aspiration for bacteriology or catheter drainage may obviate the need for difficult surgery. CT in the assessment of urinary fistula is discussed in the section on urinary tract.

In indeterminate soft-tissue masses CT can provide diagnostic information or can enable accurate biopsy.

Radiological Intervention Techniques

Needle sampling of abscess or tumour guided by ultrasound, CT or fluoroscopy is becoming commonplace. Such procedures enable accurate and prompt diagnosis and a more rational approach to medical or surgical therapy.

In relation to "pelvic congestion syndrome" there are literature reports of ovarian venography with subsequent ablation of dilated ovarian veins to good effect.

Laparoscopy

I. Rocker

The advent of fibreoptic technology provides the facility for reliable inspection of the pelvis and the anterior abdominal viscera (Table 2.7). In addition it provides the possibility of aspiration, of biopsy and of some surgical procedures. Its capacity is limited in the mid and upper abdomen but has its greatest potential in the pelvis. It is safe but must still be considered as a surgical procedure. The mortality is low (less than 1 in 10 000) and is divided between respiratory and cardiac complications and those induced by the technique, the most significant being bowel perforation. Significant morbidity totals about 1%, the majority of episodes being associated with operative rather than diagnostic laparoscopies. The problem occurs with perforation of either a viscus or a blood vessel. The problems due to diathermy burns have been reduced by safer technology and a change of tubal sterilisation technique to clip or ring occlusion rather than diathermy cauterisation. It is therefore important to realise that laparotomy may have to be performed in a small percentage of women.

The safety and reliability of laparoscopy should not encourage its use without reasonable clinical indication. At present up to 50% of diagnostic laparoscopies reveal no significant abnormality. These negative findings are important in an area with a propensity for silent disease. Good pelvic examination and an understanding of pathology is still of the utmost importance.

Not all women are suitable for laparoscopy. Poor cardiorespiratory reserve with or without obesity is a contraindication. Previous surgery, large

Table 2.7. Indications for laparoscopy

Diagnostic
Lower abdominal pain
Ectopic gestation
Pelvic inflammatory disease
Endometriosis
Ascites
Small pelvic swellings
Progress of therapy (e.g. ovarian carcinoma and endometriosis)

Surgical
Aspiration of simple cysts
Biopsy
Electrocautery or laser treatment of adhesions or endometriotic nodules

intraabdominal masses and acute peritonitis with or without bowel obstruction are also contraindications, because of the risks of visceral perforation and haemorrhage. All indications and contraindications are relative, but unless the laparoscope can be safely introduced and vision assured there is no benefit to be obtained from the procedure.

General anaesthesia is the general rule, although local anaesthesia can sometimes be used. The procedure can be undertaken as a day case or as an overnight admission, depending on local facilities. A cannula is introduced into the uterus to assist manipulation and for tubal patency testing. A carbon dioxide pneumoperitoneum is induced by transabdominal or central lower abdominal puncture. Failure to induce a pneumoperitoneum is fortunately rare. Subsequently a trocar and cannula are introduced through a 1 cm incision in the umbilical skin edge, and a laparoscope is introduced for the inspection. If necessary a probe is introduced through a second cannula to assist manipulation for clearer visualisation. Biopsy forceps, diathermy probes and scissors can also be introduced. For the more complex intrapelvic manoeuvres up to three cannulas may be inserted into the lower abdomen, so the patient should be advised of this possibility. Following completion the puncture wounds are sutured.

The immediate postoperative effects are: those associated with any general anaesthetic, shoulder pain due to subdiaphragmatic irritation by the carbon dioxide insufflated to distend the peritoneal cavity and tenderness at the puncture sites, particularly if bruising occurs. The diagnostic procedures need only a few days for recovery, but the surgical group may need 1 to 2 weeks before full activity is possible.

Management difficulties may be encountered if no pathology is detected, since not all patients will be reassured by the lack of diagnosis. In such circumstances the difficulties can be aggravated by any complications of the laparoscopy itself. It is advisable to warn patients undergoing laparoscopic sterilisation or other manipulation that laparotomy may be necessary for the safe completion of the procedure.

Hysteroscopy

Direct inspection of the uterine cavity is possible by the transcervical introduction of a narrow endoscope into the uterine cavity, which is distended with Dextran or Glycine. This can be useful in the detection of small lesions such as polyps, either endometrial or fibroid, or lost coils not visible on ultrasonography. It can also reveal the site of an early endometrial carcinoma. Its use and availability are limited but it is worth considering in women who have colicky uterine pain with some discharge or bleeding.

3 Reproduction and Pain

I. ROCKER

Preadolescence

Children under 14 years of age rarely present with lower abdominal or pelvic pain of gynaecological origin. Those who do will be suffering from one of a comparatively small group of diseases. Infection is the most likely and is limited to the vulva and vagina; although theoretically infection can ascend to involve the peritoneal cavity, this rarely happens. Infections are more common with poor hygiene and the presence of parasitic infestations. Congenital malformation of the vulva or vagina, particularly with fistula formation, prolapse of the urethral mucosa or an ectopic ureteric orifice into the vaginal vault, will predispose or mimic vaginal infections. Also the vulval and vaginal mucosae are less resistant to infection until physical maturity is achieved.

The majority of vulval or vaginal infections are non-specific, but the possibility arises of sexual abuse or of the self-introduction of foreign bodies, such as marbles, into the vagina. The presence of gonococci, chlamydia or vulval warts indicates the likelihood of sexual activity or, more significantly, of sexual abuse. There is the suggestion that abuse in childhood predisposes to the development of chronic pelvic pain in adulthood.

The history is usually presented by the mother but if presented by the father without the mother should sound a warning note of a higher likelihood of sexual abuse. This does not, however, imply that fathers are not concerned about their daughters. The complaint is of an excessive vaginal discharge or vulval and perineal reddening and swelling, which results in discomfort in micturition or defaecation, sleeplessness or irritability. Febrile illness is rarely described, the infant or child being able to continue in playschool or primary school. The first or second infection may resolve spontaneously with local bathing, particularly if there is no vaginitis. Subsequent episodes will be presented to the family practitioner, who will have to balance the benefit of a complete examination against the drawbacks of pelvic examination and admission to hospital of a 4- or 5-year-old child. A total examination will include vulval inspection and palpation, rectal examination and vaginal inspection with a 3–4 mm endoscope. The history is the guide to the degree of examination needed. A short history of recurrent infection and a negative abdominal and vulval inspection without evidence of gross oedema, purulent exudate or tenderness, and clean urethral, vaginal and anal orifices requires a simple bacteriological smear and culture. Non-specific organisms such as streptococci and staphylococci account for the majority of infections. Monilia may be the result of antibiotic therapy for infection at other sites. Diabetes in this age group is likely to have a more acute onset associated with general illness or a severe infection. The discovery of gonococci or trichomonas will necessitate a complete examination, because the possibility of sexual abuse has to be excluded. Chlamydia will not be discovered on routine bacteriological examination. A suspicion of a foreign body arises if there is more vaginitis than vulvitis. Visual anomalies of the vulvo-vagina-perineal area or a protuberant urethral mucosa will indicate the need for a full examination under anaesthesia. Recurrent nose and throat infections may also result in digital transfer of infection to the vagina. The possibility of skin allergies or eczema should be considered, and recurrent infections may be the prodromal phase of skin dystrophies such as lichen sclerosis.

Examination is best performed in the presence of the mother. If sexual abuse is suspected by history or circumstance, then it is preferable that the examination be performed by a paediatrician or gynaecologist with specific experience. Assurance that no painful procedure is to be undertaken and allowing the child to see the size of the bacteriological swab should permit stage A examination (Table 3.1) to be completed. For a fuller examination

Table 3.1. Examination of vulvovaginitis

Stage A
Abdominal examination:
　Local inspection and palpation:
　　part labia to inspect introitus and urethra
　　part buttock to inspect anus
　Swab from vulva and or introitus – smear
　Stool for worms
　Mid-stream urine

Stage B
Examination under anaesthesia:
　rectal
　vaginal in older children using "little" finger
Inspection of vagina and cervix
Vaginal and cervical secretions:
　bacteriological culture (see Table 2.6, p. 41)
　saline suspension for sperm detection
Vaginal/cervical smears
Vaginal biopsy if history of diethylstilboestrol in pregnancy
Vulval biopsy if dystrophy suspected
Nasal/throat swab if recurrent infections

the child should be referred to a paediatrician rather than a general gynaecologist. Management of secondary infection caused by a foreign body in the vagina is self-evident. Recurrence after removal of the object is unlikely. The main group with staphylococcal and particularly coliform infection need careful instruction in personal hygiene, directed to the prevention of vulval soiling following defaecation. Oestrogen cream can be helpful in the under 7s, but long term use is to be avoided. A course for 3 to 4 weeks is unlikely to produce an oestrogenising effect on the breast, but for recurrent infections full investigation needs to be repeated. Labial adhesion is a problem in that it produces an abnormal appearance of the vulva, but delicate lateral pressure on the skin reveals the paper-thin film which adjoins the opposing labial folds. Although the division of the adhesion is simple, it is painful and best performed under anaesthesia. This will reveal a surface desquamation but without any significant underlying vaginitis. Following division, the mother should be instructed to pay regular attention to the vulva so that readhesion does not occur. Gentle separation once a week following a bath is probably all that is required. If it recurs, then some oestrogen cream can be helpful until sexual maturity has been achieved.

Trauma

Trauma results from accidents whilst riding bicycles or playing on swings or any activity in which the child can fall astride a bar or solid ridge. The acute phase produces laceration, haematoma formation and oedema. If extended to the urethra, retention of urine can occur. If not diagnosed then the subsequent disfiguration or stenosis of the urethra can present with recurrent episodes of urinary difficulties, frequency and on occasion incontinence. All vulvovaginal haematomas may result in abscess formation and primary drainage has to be considered. It is also important to reassure the parents, if no significant damage has occurred, that the injury is unlikely to affect future reproductive development.

In a 14-year-old sexual activity, whether by abuse or by consent, may result in vulvovaginal laceration. Healed small hymenal defects alone are not indicative of sexual activity; it is the extent and appearance of the defect in relation to age that will give the clue. The less mature vaginal mucosa is more prone to laceration and to inflammatory reaction. A ragged hymen and an open vulva in a 6 to 8 year old are obviously suspect. A balanced suspicion of human nature and a critical appraisal of physical signs will guide accurate diagnosis and management. The management of sex abuse requires a multidisciplinary approach, and all health authorities should have this facility. A preliminary assessment should include a second opinion. Indication for admission following sexual or non-sexual trauma will depend on the visible extent of the lesion and the degree of bleeding and pain. A small vulval laceration does not exclude vaginal or vault laceration, and a blood clot of several centimetres in diameter should warn of the possibility of internal trauma.

Congenital Malformations

Congenital malformations of the cloaca and urogenital sinus in the extreme form are likely to have been discovered in the neonate, particularly if there is any problem of micturition or defaecation. Problems presenting in the postneonatal period include an ectopic ureter, whose leakage will present in those who are not dry by 2 to 3 years of age. Their incontinence will continue day and night, and even intravenous pyelography may fail to detect the ectopic siting of the ureteric orifice. This has been described in various positions of the anterior or lateral vagina and vaginal vault. Congenital sagittal malformations of the vagina do not predispose to any significant problem in this young age group. A transverse septum is of considerable importance because, if it is complete, it will give rise to a haematocolpos which can present either as an acute swelling or as acute or recurrent pain. It must not be confused with an absent vagina in association with normal female chromosomes or with vaginal aplasia in intersex or testicular feminisation syndromes.

Congenital anomalies of the uterus are of wide range, from a bicornuate uterus and cervix through all combinations of uterine shape and conjoined cervices to complete dual uterocervicovaginal systems. The more complete the bifid defect, the less likely there are to be pathological problems, though many problems of interpretation, particularly in pregnancy, can arise. Cervical atresia is rare and is likely to present as a haematometra. The anomalies of the uterus and vagina have significant association with renal abnormality, which can be detected by intravenous pyelography. Such examination can be delayed until later life unless there is a history of renal tract infection. It is most important to communicate clearly the "normality" of the majority of these manifestations and to instil confidence in future feminine capacity.

Cysts and Tumours

Foetal ovarian cysts can now be discovered in utero by ultrasonography. Formerly such cysts would be discovered only if they were 8–10 cm in diameter and either visible or palpable abdominally at delivery. In infancy, ovarian follicular cysts are the most likely, and these can be removed with ovarian conservation. However, scanning can give such clear pictures that, in a case of intrauterine discovery, follow-up is required rather than immediate surgery. The majority of the cysts are of a simple serous type and will, if big enough, cause lower abdominal discomfort. But, as with the adult, they are more likely to present because of secondary symptoms such as urinary or faecal disturbance. A follicular cyst may produce sufficient oestrogen to cause precocious development. Some 25%–30% of ovarian tumours are malignant and range from granulosa cell (oestrogen secreting) to arrhenoblastoma (androgen secreting) tumours. The presentation is usually that of a fit child with vague lower abdominal pressure symptoms and a palpable abdominal swelling, which may be massive in relation to the child's overall size. The hormonal functioning malignant tumours are more likely to present with the additional general debility. Should surgical castration be necessary then the discussion should include long term support, particularly with regard to secondary sexual development.

Vulva and Vagina

Benign paraurethral cysts, Gartnerian remnants, cysts of the lateral vaginal wall and vulval cysts occur. They vary in size and are significant if disturbing micturition. Malignancy in the form of a mixed mesodermal tumour (sarcoma botyroides) and clear-cell carcinoma following stilboestrol in pregnancy will cause both discharge and bleeding.

The Cervix

The cervix can be associated with benign granulomatous polyps, condylomata and childhood carcinoma of the cervix. The uterine corpus has an extremely rare record of malignancy. The cervical lesions are likely to give rise to vaginal discharge and some degree of bleeding and this sequence of events should entail a full examination.

Dysmenorrhoea

Primary or spasmodic dysmenorrhoea is an ill-defined syndrome in relation to its aetiology but not in presentation. It starts within a few months of, and up to 5 or more years after, the onset of menstruation and, in the younger age group, once an ovulatory pattern has been established. In the early teens, some 5% of youngsters suffer, but the figure goes up to 25% of women by their late teens. Only a small percentage are totally incapacitated.

Dysmenorrhoea in a girl is closely related to her mother's experience of the same discomfort. The cause is not specifically known, but possible causes are listed in Table 3.2. There is no convincing evidence that cervical obstruction or uterine hypoplasia or anomaly is a significant factor. Neither can psychoneurosis be considered as a cause of primary dysmenorrhoea. There is an understandable correlation between reactive anxiety and recurrent pain. Neurogenic pain threshold is a possible factor in a small group of young women. The older theories suggested myometrial ischaemia, muscle tracings showing a changing disorderly pattern of contraction and a higher level of uterine tonus in sufferers with dysmenorrhoea. Uterine activity is related to hormone levels and hormone balance, but these are not considered to be the direct cause. There is also a relation between

Table 3.2. Causes of dysmenorrhoea

Mechanical obstruction:
 cervical
 uterine hypoplasia
 uterine anomalies (congenital)

Myometrial activity:
 ischaemia
 myometrial spasm
Neurological
Psychological
Hormonal imbalance
Prostaglandin

hormone production, hormone balance and prostaglandins. Prostaglandins $F_{2\alpha}$ and E_2 are raised in women with dysmenorrhoea. The correlation of prostaglandin, oestrogen and progesterone balance and muscular activity are well described and reflect the symptoms of spasmodic dysmenorrhoea. Pain itself is a correlation of various symptoms, from cultural or psychosexual to neuroanatomical response.

The younger the patient the more likely she is to be accompanied by her mother or an aunt. An independent history may be difficult to obtain tactfully, but the attempt is worth while. Similarly for a girl attending on her own, no suggestion should be made of consultation with her parents without her consent. This allows a position of trust to be established and enables the doctor to assess the patient as fully as possible without the need for laboratory technology.

The lower abdominal pain of dysmenorrhoea starts a few hours before or during the first few hours of menstruation. It may spread into both iliac fossae and down the inner aspects of the thighs and also involve the sacral area. The pain is spasmodic and colicky, each spasm lasting from a few to many minutes but with an underlying abdominal and sacral discomfort remaining. It can be associated with malaise, prostration, vomiting, diarrhoea, and fainting. A peak of pain and associated effects is reached after 3 to 4 hours and is usually resolved within 24 hours. There is no absolute timing, but symptoms of longer duration should be a cause for concern, lest the presentation is secondary to pelvic pathology. Examination of the abdomen does not usually suggest intraperitoneal irritation, nor are there any general signs of fever, significant tachycardia or change in blood pressure. It is therefore the history and the absence of pelvic physical signs that provide the basis for diagnosis.

The true incidence of primary dysmenorrhoea is unknown as the lesser degrees are accepted by both public and profession as being within normal limits. This results in under-reporting or in self-treatment. The history is classic, and physical examination is negative. Girls of 16 and over can usually be examined vaginally, and the palpation of a normal vagina and uterus is a reassuring beginning for counselling. If a satisfactory pelvic examination is impossible or deemed inadvisable, then high-resolution pelvic ultrasonography can outline the uterus and the ovaries, but the radiologist must be aware of this requirement. Examination under anaesthesia and laparoscopy are reserved for the severe and non-responding cases.

Difficulties of management arise if a diagnosis is incorrect or if there is distrust, poor communication and any underlying fears or ignorance about menstruation which are not elucidated. The majority of attenders seek reassurance that there is no evidence of disease. It is important to know the details of lifestyle and the degree to which dysmenorrhoea frustrates it. In many cases it is the fear of such a possibility that leads to consultation. Similarly, concern about examinations, holidays or approaching marriage may provide the impetus to seek help. It is therefore important to have a constructive attitude to the diagnosis and treatment and to recognise that dysmenorrhoea is a complex problem, no single treatment being totally effective.

The first line of management is of relaxed counselling and simple analgesia. It is likely that such drugs have been used before attendance. For patients with a regular cycle, pre-emptive treatment commencing 24 to 48 hours before the onset of menstruation is worth trying. It is important to explain that no method of treatment can be guaranteed to provide immediate and complete relief and therefore various analgesics should be tried (Table 3.3).

Time should be given to ensure that the patient understands menstruation and to answer queries as to future effects. The complex interrelationship of adolescence, femininity and family require understanding and intuition at the consultation.

Advice that the pain will improve after pregnancy and labour may have some foundation in fact but is of poor prognostic accuracy. The understanding that physical disease will not be overlooked and that there is a wide range of supportive treatment should be ensured. Aspirin, paracetamol and the antiprostaglandins are all likely to be effective, and the aim should be for maximum relief with minimal side-effects. Guidance should be given as to the gastrointestinal disturbances of dyspepsia, particularly nausea and diarrhoea, the central nervous effects of headache and irritability and allergic effects such as bronchospasm. In long-term use the possibilities of renal effect and blood dyscrasia should be recorded on the notes for regular assessment.

Hormonal preparations are extremely effective, and with the increasing interest in the long-term effects of breast, ovarian and cervical cancer, such queries should be answered directly with the information that is at present available. In essence, combined pill use may be associated with an increase in breast and cervical cancer in later life and a reduction of ovarian malignancy. The changing risk is small, particularly for short-term use of less than 1 to 2 years.

Table 3.3. Management of dysmenorrhoea

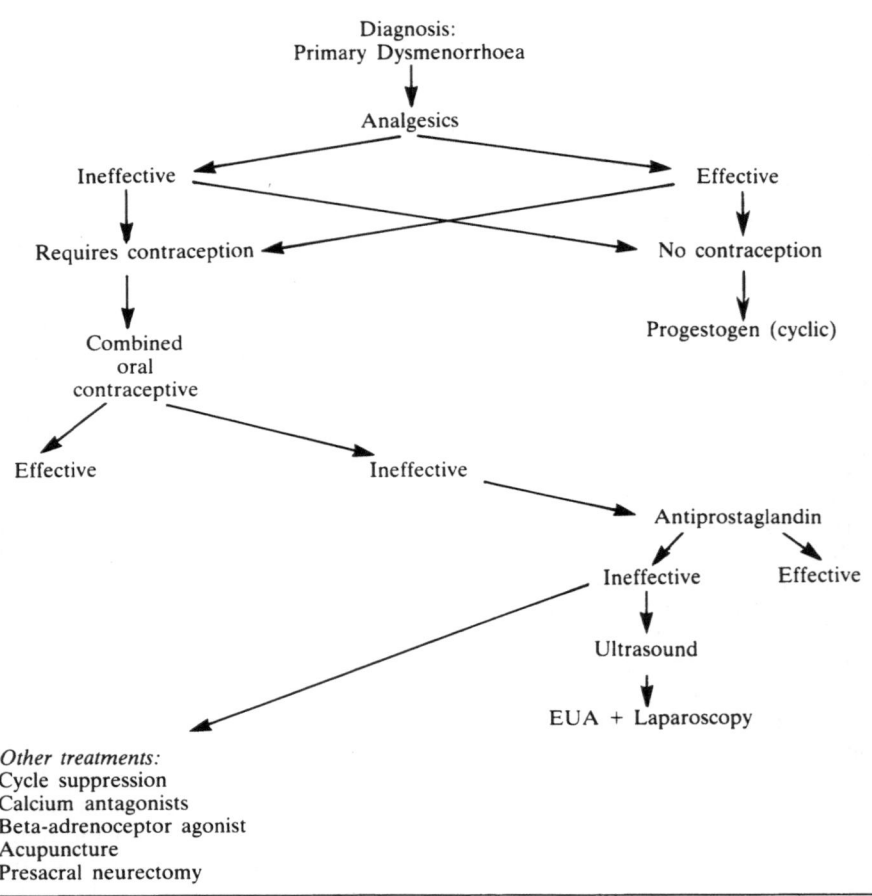

EUA, examination under anaesthesia.

For those who want contraception, the combined oral contraceptive will effectively stop dysmenorrhoea in up to 80% of cases. The decision to use the combined pill in young teenagers can usually be resolved by frank discussion with patient and parents (the latter only with the patient's consent). The best results are likely to be obtained in girls who undertake therapy and guidance willingly. The lower-dose contraceptive pills do not necessarily prevent follicle production, and therefore one of the medium-dose pills is preferable, utilising 30–35 μg ethinyl oestradiol and 1 mg of norethisterone or an equivalent dose of the new progestogens. A trial of at least 3 months is required, and some patients may wish to use this form of therapy intermittently. However, it is not suitable for a single month of treatment. Duration of use is negotiable but is likely to continue until the girl is in her early twenties or wants to conceive.

For those who do not wish to use the combined pill, progestogens may be equally effective. There are a small number who will respond to progestogen alone when the combined oestrogen/progestogen pill has failed and vice versa.

The derivatives of natural progesterone, such as dyhydrogesterone, or of testosterone or norethisterone are the most commonly used. Theoretically any of the progestogens is effective but the progesterone derivatives are less likely to be virilising. The dose regimen is from the 5th to the 25th day of the cycle and may be used successfully for many years. Because of its interrupted 21-day usage it is not suitable for contraception.

If analgesics alone or hormone preparations alone do not bring about sufficient relief then it is reasonable to combine these therapies, but if significant improvement is not obtained then diagnostic review is mandatory. At this stage a decision has to be made whether the indications are for physical assessment (mainly of scanning, examination under anaesthesia and laparoscopy) or for psychological review. Requests for hypnotherapy, acupuncture or transcutaneous nerve stimulation should be considered if available.

Cycle suppression for up to 3 months will be helpful during examinations and in the early weeks of marriage and is on occasion used as a diagnostic test. Norethisterone 10–20 mg daily or medroxyprogesterone 30–40 mg daily will inhibit menstruation, although there is the risk of weight gain and breakthrough bleeding. The latter risk can be reduced if the progestogen dosage is increased stepwise at intervals of 3 to 4 weeks. The anti-oestrogen danazol at a dose of 600–800 mg daily can also inhibit menstruation but is more likely to have the side-effect of weight gain and greasy skin with occasionally acne-like rashes. The gonadotrophin releasing analogue buserelin can also produce a temporary artificial menopause. It is, however, an expensive form of treatment and requires either daily injection or intranasal application five times daily. Side-effects such as hot flushes may also occur. It is therefore best reserved for a particular occasion, but the knowledge that such temporary treatment is available is in itself helpful.

There have been reports that calcium antagonists such as nifedipine 20–40 mg orally will reduce myometrial activity within 10 to 30 minutes. Similarly, terbutaline sulphate intravenously 0.25–0.5 mg will alleviate dysmenorrhoea for 1 to 2 hours. Both drugs have concomitant effects of tachycardia, flushes and headache. Such treatment has not been widely used but may be a useful emergency treatment.

Presacral neurectomy can be effective if sufficient fibres of the presacral plexus can be divided. Before laparoscopy became available, the laparotomy was also diagnostic. The operation has risks, including menorrhagia and a failure rate related to selection and poor guidelines. Because of the poor results it is now rarely performed. It should therefore be considered only for the rare persistent and intractable case of dysmenorrhoea.

The cornerstone of management remains accurate diagnosis and giving the patient an opportunity for private discussion. This should also remove fears about menstruation, e.g., dirty blood, and so provide an educational input. Analgesics, steroid hormones and antiprostaglandins are the basics of the drug armamentarium. Patients in whom psychoneurosis is evident or the condition has produced a severe reactive anxiety state should be encouraged to seek psychological counselling.

Sexual Activity and Pelvic Pain

A woman's ability to engage in intravaginal coitus may not be accompanied by a wish to do so, and this can produce a dilemma which persists as a clinical problem of sexual difficulty and pain. Education and expectation are significant partners. Personal experience, both familial and extrafamilial, are dominant factors, but experiences of childhood or adult abuse may never come to the surface. For this reason empirical treatment is unlikely to succeed. Sexual knowledge, hopes, fears and fantasies are daily transmitted by books, magazines and television. In adolescence and in early womanhood the knowledge of pelvic inflammatory disease, sexually transmitted disease and cervical dysplasia all add to the factors that influence attitudes. Unwelcome coitus can therefore produce a sensation of pressure which is painful and bladder pressure giving rise to urgency. Simplistic sensory physiological reasoning is just the beginning of understanding the problem of diagnosis and management. It is often unwise to try and obtain a relevant history at the first consultation.

Dyspareunia

Vaginal and pelvic pain associated with willing participation in heterosexual activity can be approached on the basis of primary and secondary dyspareunia. The primary causes of introital dyspareunia are rarely due to anatomical malformation but probably result from infection or poor coital technique. The secondary causes are most commonly perineal laceration or incision associated with childbirth and, in later life, vulval atrophy. Vulval skin disease such as lichen sclerosis will reduce natural elasticity and in its early stages will show little visible evidence. This lesion can occur in childhood but is much more common postmenopausally. Vulval atrophy produces loss of subcutaneous tissue in the fourchette, resulting in a tissue web which becomes the posterior wall of the introitus. A previous perineorrhaphy can produce a similar effect.

The degree of pain will affect the action of the levatores ani, which if contracted will close the vagina and produce vaginismus. Introital pain and vaginismus are due to a combination of ignorance, fear and poor coital-technique.

Forced intercourse or rape will be a single event with bruising and laceration of varying degree which, if superficial, will heal in about 10 days.

A youngster may present with inability to introduce a tampon for menstrual hygiene. Without overcoming anatomical ignorance and understandable fear, the problem will progress. The woman complaining of introital dyspareunia without obvious visible or palpable anomaly is likely to have a deeper psychological problem. Discussion of such problems and of coital technique is best undertaken by practitioners who have had the requisite training. Such expertise will be found in family planning, psychiatric and less frequently in gynaecological clinics. For the young it is important not to aggravate the problem by suggesting that the vagina is too small. Training in the use of vaginal dilators can be crude therapy and should not be attempted if a one-finger vaginal examination cannot be performed or the woman is reluctant and unable to introduce her own finger into her vagina. The small group for whom surgery is indicated are found to have a marked hymen with a superior edge reaching the external urethral meatus. The group in whom dyspareunia prevents coitus with or without vaginismus is distinct and needs specialist psychosexual management. The group who maintain intravaginal coitus but with discomfort are more likely to have a discoverable cause. Fear of pregnancy is still a common complaint even if unvoiced, but marriage, social and financial problems or direct unhappy experience of pregnancy or an indirect family experience may be the cause of lack of relaxation or lack of libido which will be expressed as painful coitus. Anatomical problems due to uterine prolapse or retroversion of the uterus are discussed on pp. 105–108. Pelvic disease, inflammatory, neoplastic, endometriotic and postsurgical causes of dyspareunia are discussed in the relevant sections.

Pregnancy

Pregnancy is associated with major physiological and anatomical changes in the pelvis and the abdomen. Following fertilisation of the ovum the residual follicle continues to enlarge and becomes the functioning corpus luteum. This enlargement doubles the volume of the ovary within 2 to 3 weeks. The uterus rapidly increases in size and by the 8th week will fill most of the upper half of the pelvic cavity, and in thin women the fundus is readily palpable just above the symphysis pubi. These changes are associated with a marked increase of blood flow in the ovarian and uterine vessels and the size of these vessels, particularly within the broad ligament. Retroversion of the uterus is present in 10% of women, and in an additional 10% retroversion occurs during early pregnancy. In both groups spontaneous correction to anteversion occurs between the 10th and 12th weeks of pregnancy. The enlarging uterus impinges on the bladder, resulting in frequency of micturition. The retroflexed uterus causes a lesser effect on the rectum. The rare circumstance of an impacted retroverted uterus will produce acute onset of urinary retention, and the severe pain that occurs with the first phase of total urinary retention is commonly preceded by urinary discomfort. Pelvic discomfort in early pregnancy is of minor degree, but if pain is significant an abnormality of pregnancy or concurrent disease has to be considered.

In the earlier part of the second trimester, between the 13th and 20th weeks, the uterus is out of the pelvis and in the lower abdomen and causes few pressure effects. The pelvic girdle is accommodating to the ligamentous relaxation that takes place, so that sacroiliac discomfort is more common. The symphysis pubis is not a cause of physiological discomfort, and any pain in that area should be considered pathological.

The majority or early pregnancies are diagnosed by amenorrhoea of 6 to 8 weeks' duration and a positive pregnancy test. The secondary signs of nausea, frequency of micturition and breast tenderness are of lesser importance. The place of bimanual examination of the pelvis has been eroded by ultrasound scanning but should still be performed. Without such clinical information management of problems associated with pain becomes more difficult. Fig. 3.1 shows a pregnancy in the left side of a double uterus.

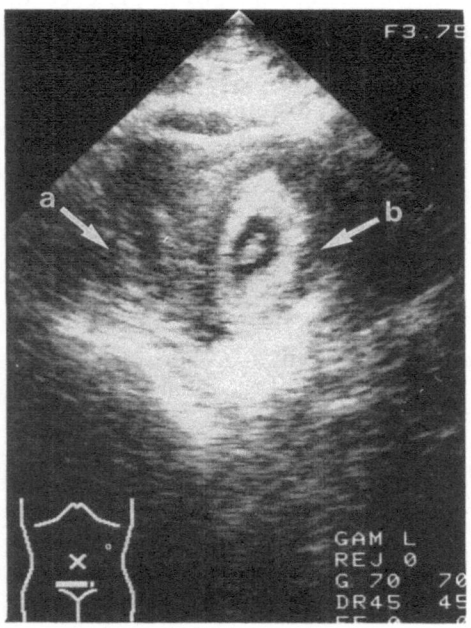

Fig. 3.1. Double uterus showing pregnancy in the left side: **a**, non-pregnant right uterus; **b**, pregnant left uterus.

Pelvic examination may be ill-advised or refused by virtue of a woman's culture or personal experience. Ethnic susceptibility is well recognised, and examination by a female doctor only will often be permitted. The most common cause for refusal is experience of a previous miscarriage, and in this circumstance only a commonsense decision is possible. The medical viewpoint is that pelvic examination will not induce miscarriage, and if this explanation is not acceptable then ultrasound scanning will usually be agreed. A smaller group is associated with previous psychosexual problems and needs careful reappraisal of the history and discussion of management in pregnancy and labour.

The physiological discomforts of pregnancy are well recognised and are part of discussion that should have taken place either before conception or in early pregnancy.

To communicate that pain is part of pregnancy is unwise and will limit the patient's confidence if pathological events are subsequently found. Pain of varying degree will be present in the miscarriage of intrauterine pregnancy, in molar changes in pregnancy and in ectopic pregnancy. It will be associated with previous gynaecological problems such as fibroids and ovarian cysts and with other acute or chronic lower pelvic pathology.

Uterine Contractility and Labour

The uterine muscle contracts throughout pregnancy, the pattern being irregular and not associated with cervical dilatation. Uterine contractility at the 6th week of pregnancy has been described and is utilised as a diagnostic sign of pregnancy, but there is no specific pattern of frequency of duration or degree and it is rarely noted by the pregnant woman before the 32nd week of pregnancy. The gradual increase in frequency of contractions, which will culminate in a regular pattern, is taken as a good sign for future normal uterine function in labour. The 28th week of gestation is taken to be the earliest date of premature labour, but in practice this is an artificial division. The reality is whether independent foetal life can be maintained. The cause of primary or idiopathic premature uterine activity is not known in any trimester of pregnancy. Secondary activity is associated with trophoblastic or placental disruption or cessation of function and can occasionally be due to trauma or induced by oxytocic drugs.

A number of conditions are associated with premature labour, namely, congenital abnormalities of the uterus, twin pregnancy, foetal anomalies (particularly with polyhydramnios), maternal pyrexia due to infections or intrauterine foetal death. The problem is one of foetal viability (unless associated with placental abruption) or maternal infection of such a degree that foetal and maternal risk are interrelated.

Lower abdominal pain, with or without backache, that has persisted for a few hours requires assessment. Most commonly it is not an additional feature to maternal illness. In the absence of bleeding and cervical dilatation it is important to decide whether discomfort or pain with associated uterine contractility is a prodromal phase of idiopathic or secondary miscarriage prior to 28 weeks or labour. The diagnostic problem is not acute in pregnancies of 34 or more weeks if it is due to the onset of labour and not to placental disruption. The diagnosis and management of miscarriage is described on p. 73, but many features are similar, namely, uterine contraction with uterine tenderness, particularly if localised bleeding and cervical dilatation become the criteria for diagnosis. Anxiety will enhance the severity of presentation, but a few hours will often determine the diagnosis, because progressive severity will make it more likely that labour will ensue. Bedside diagnosis has to determine whether or not hospital admission is indicated. A non-tender uterus without irritability on pressure and without contraction, with good foetal movement and foetal heart sounds does not warrant urgent admission. An irritable and/or tender uterus particularly if localised needs constant assessment and requires transfer to a specialised obstetric unit.

There is therefore a group of women presenting with a diagnosis of spurious labour who may be admitted several times during the course of pregnancy to their obstetric unit. Even with modern technology it may be impossible to decide whether the situation is truly idiopathic and that any foetal problems of labour will be solely of prematurity or whether there is a possibility of intermittent placental disruption with possible anoxia. Management is decided by foetal age and maternal risk. Such definition is complex, but in clinical practice foetal age is grouped at 26 to 29 weeks, 30 to 33 weeks and 34 weeks onwards. If the cause of premature labour is impending placental failure, then prevention with drugs such as salbutamol and ritrodine may reduce the chance of survival. Drug inhibition of labour is not at present a reliable technology, and there is therefore a wide variation of practice. Clinical experience is still a cardinal factor despite tocography and ultrasonography.

The possibility of premature labour is an indication for admission to an obstetric unit with the necessary intensive care facilities for the premature baby. The decision about how to manage labour is still unresolved though there is increasing tendency to use Caesarean section. A practicable outline protocol is one which allows for vaginal deliveries in the 34-week group unless foetal distress ensues. A bias towards Caesarean section is greatest at the 28th week and reduces with increasing foetal age and maturity. Suppression of pain is secondary to diagnosis; in the non-pathological group relief of anxiety and explanation that the uterus can contract spontaneously and will do so in response to pressure is all that may be required. The use of beta-sympathomimetic drugs, ethyl alcohol or antiprostaglandins is an individual decision but discussion before such usage should include the problems of diagnosis and the merits and demerits of Caesarean section.

The Ovary in Pregnancy

The ovary, having discharged its ovum, will progress to form a corpus luteum if fertilisation and implantation take place. The ovary becomes enlarged and the enlargement is a useful secondary sign of pregnancy.

Discomfort occurs if the enlargement is unusually great, if the vascularity of the vessels in the broad ligament is increased or if pressure is enhanced by an association with uterine retroversion. Modern technology aggravates this problem if at ultrasonography the anechoic area in the ovary is considered to be a true, if small, cyst. A palpable ovary in the first trimester of pregnancy is therefore not of pathological significance even if enlarged to 4–5 cm in diameter. As the uterus rises out of the pelvis the ovary becomes impalpable but is usually 4–5 cm away from the lateral edge of the uterus.

Slight bleeding or blood transudation from a corpus luteum will irritate the pelvic peritoneum and produce a syndrome of amenorrhoea, enlarged uterus, pain and tenderness which mimics an ectopic gestation. There is, however, no uterine bleeding unless there is an associated threat of miscarriage. A complete rupture of the corpus luteum produces an acute emergency which can be resolved by a laparotomy. Oophorectomy should not be necessary. Resuturing the bleeding edge of a corpus luteum is difficult because of the fragility of the tissues, but total removal of the corpus luteum and obliteration of the ovarian cavity can be performed. The closer to 12 weeks' gestation the lesser the risk of miscarriage.

Torsion of the pedicle of an enlarged ovary can occur, particularly on the side containing a corpus luteum, and will produce an acute syndrome with backache and sudden vomiting in addition to the lower abdominal pain. The pain will tend to be localised to one or other side of the lower abdomen with tenderness and guarding as well as amenorrhoea and the enlarged pregnant uterus. This is an acute emergency, which will require salpingo-oophorectomy.

Abnormalities of Intrauterine Pregnancy

Pregnancy failure will involve pain due to the haemorrhagic disruption of trophoblast or placenta and/or the uterine contractions that are associated. Some 14% of women miscarry between the 6th and 28th week of pregnancy, and 4%–6% of women labour prematurely. Approximately 8% of first-trimester pregnancy failures are associated with a blighted ovum, which is diagnosable by the 6th week. In the majority of cases miscarriage will take place by the 8th week of amenorrhoea. 25%–50% of pregnancies fail before 6 weeks, but such early failure is unlikely to cause pelvic pain. Very early miscarriage is usually considered to be an unusually painful or prolonged menstruation. Though early miscarriage is heralded by bleeding and then pain, the sequence may last from 1 day to several weeks, particularly in the case of "missed" abortion. In 60%–80% of earlier miscarriages a developmental error has occurred, but without special techniques such as chromosome analysis the cause is unlikely to be established.

There is therefore a pregnancy failure with prior or subsequent trophoblast separation over a time scale usually no longer than 2 weeks. Non-expulsion of pregnancy tissue is associated with the syndrome of missed abortion and partial expulsion that of incomplete miscarriage.

In the majority of miscarriages the presenting sign is bleeding, and management depends on the degree of bleeding and on the state of the cervix and uterine size. At one end of the spectrum will be a tightly closed cervix and a uterine body of size equivalent to the duration of amenorrhoea. At the other end of the spectrum will be a uterus smaller in size, a widely opened cervix and blood clot and extruded pregnancy tissue in the vault of the vagina. Immersion of blood clot in cold water will allow separation into decidual and trophoblastic solid tissue and dissolved blood, so establishing whether there is any likelihood of a pregnancy being maintained. Before 10 weeks a foetus is rarely recognised. The presence of vesicles will necessitate histological examination to exclude the diagnosis of hydatidiform mole. The smaller group with lesser bleeding, longer duration of amenorrhoea and pain will be associated with a closed cervix and a firmer uterus but the presence and viability of a foetus can be determined ultrasonically, by auscultation of the foetal heart or visually by foetal form and movement. Urinary pregnancy tests are now quick and highly sensitive but may remain weakly positive even if foetal death has just occurred because of the presence of excreted gonadotrophin in the bladder urine. Modern technology provides an immediate answer but not necessarily an accurate forecast of subsequent survival. Management must therefore include an awareness of the emotional problems associated with pregnancy and the guilt feelings that may be present because of lifestyle. Care should be taken before endorsing physical or sexual activity as a cause of miscarriage. Public awareness of miscarriage risks make it advisable to include bacteriological examination for the possibility of a cause such as listeriosis.

Trophoblastic Disease

Trophoblastic disease ranges from the benign hydatidiform mole to the rare but highly invasive chorion carcinoma. The development of abnormal trophoblast without a foetus results in rapid growth of the uterus and ovaries and an exaggeration of secondary pregnancy characteristics. The ovaries contain multiple theca luteal cysts, which are thin walled and liable to rupture. The uterus becomes diffusely enlarged and tender if intrauterine bleeding has occurred. Excessive nausea and vomiting and symptoms and signs suggestive of pre-eclampsia are common. The condition does have a tissue marker, namely, the level of chorionic gonadotrophin, which can be assessed quantitatively in blood and urine. Ultrasound visualisation reveals the classic multiechoic appearance, which is accurately diagnostic. This combination allows early diagnosis, thereby preventing the woman becoming seriously ill and distraught with exaggerated symptoms of pregnancy, avoiding pain from an overdistended uterus and lower abdomen, and reducing the risk of haemorrhage at evacuation of the trophoblast from the uterus.

The diagnosis would usually have been made because a woman with excessive vomiting, early onset of hypertension and a uterus larger than the expected date of pregnancy would develop lower abdominal pain and bleeding. Ultrasonography will show the multiple vesicles of hydatidiform degeneration. A smaller group will present with the pain and intermittent bleeding, the uterus not having a significant discrepancy in size, in whom qualitative pregnancy tests may encourage conservative management to maintain pregnancy. Measurement of gonadotrophin level and ultrasonography provide the diagnosis.

Vacuum aspiration of the uterine contents is the preferred method. This reduces the risk of haemorrhage and of embolisation of a trophoblast tissue. Total clearance may not be achieved at the first attempt, because the trophoblastic tissue may remain embedded in the uterine muscle. Histology and gonadotrophin output will determine the division into the main subgroups, the largest being those with hydatidiform mole, in which regression will occur within 6 months. The next group are those with a slow fall of gonadotrophin levels which have to be treated with chemotherapy on the same regimen as the rarer chorioncarcinoma. The third group are those whose rising gonadotrophin levels and intrauterine changes or secondary deposits of chorioncarcinoma necessitate intensive combined treatment. This is best undertaken at a regional specialist unit.

Communication in this condition is difficult, since couples do not readily comprehend that a placenta can grow without formation of a foetus. Without this understanding, the necessary discussion explaining the need for follow-up for 2 years with blood and urinary gonadotrophin assay is difficult. The purpose of follow-up is to detect residual trophoblast and prevent chorioncarcinoma, and this must be carefully explained. Women who need pre-emptive chemotherapy must be reassured that cure and subsequent pregnancy are possible. In the 90% with benign hydatidiform moles normal pregnancy is the rule following completion of surveillance. The combined contraceptive pill is not advisable in the follow-up phase as it slows the fall of chorionic gonadotrophin levels. Removal of fear is therefore an important part of management.

Ectopic Gestation

Ectopic gestation occurs in about 1 in 200 of all pregnancies and is virtually always in the Fallopian tube. The majority of ectopic gestations have been diagnosed by the 10th week of pregnancy. Pathological changes and timing are related to the site of implantation, so that isthmial pregnancy will result in recurrent colicky pain by the 5th or 6th week, whereas ampullary implantation may not produce pain until intraperitoneal bleeding has occurred. Trophoblastic and foetal death will mimic the changes of a missed intrauterine abortion, so that severe or acute pain does not occur. The range extends from an unruptured ectopic with extrusion of a tubal mole through the ampullary end with little bleeding or minor discomfort to (most commonly) a gestation sac distending the tube, slight intraperitoneal leaking through the ampulla, subsequent rupture of the gestation sac into the uterine cavity and foetal death with the passage of a uterine decidual cast. Abdominal and pelvic pain are related to the amount of bleeding into the peritoneal cavity, each bolus of blood producing pain for some 12 to 24 hours. The passage of blood to the paracolic gutter of the subdiaphragm gives rise to shoulder pain. In addition there are the changes of shock, which are related to the rate of loss and the total volume of blood loss. In 10% of cases the classic presentation of ectopic gestation presents as an acute abdominal emergency due to intraperitoneal haemorrhage. Immediate laparatomy is then mandatory.

Ectopic pregnancy produces amenorrhoea, bleeding, pelvic pain and tenderness of an extrauterine swelling. The diagnosis is based on suspicion, particularly for women using a progestational contraceptive, or an intrauterine contraceptive device or those with previous pelvic inflammatory disease, particularly with reconstructive surgery.

Clinical examination elicits lower abdominal pain, pelvic tenderness and guarding and rebound tenderness. The uterus is firm and smaller than the duration of amenorrhoea would suggest. Pelvic tenderness can be so severe as to inhibit a complete examination. Gently performed, examination will outline an extrauterine swelling which is acutely tender and does not have readily demarcated margins. The beta subunit of human chorionic gonadotrophin is a useful diagnostic aid in the early cases if the result is readily available. Ultrasonography will provide supportive evidence that no intrauterine pregnancy exists and that there may be a swelling on the site of the Fallopian tube and the presence of blood in the pouch of Douglas. Coexistent intrauterine and tubal pregnancy has always to be considered. Laparoscopy will reveal the tubal changes and the blood in the pelvic cavity. It can, however, be unreliable before the 6th week of gestation.

The cornerstone of management is early diagnosis, which reduces the risk of haemorrhage and of surgery and the later problems of pelvic infection resulting from incomplete intraperitoneal lavage. Partial salpingectomy to control haemorrhage is the usual operation. Immediate tubal reconstruction causes an even higher risk of subsequent ectopic pregnancy but may have to be considered when the operation is being performed on a woman with only a single Fallopian tube. The first phase is therefore accurate diagnosis and laparotomy to prevent massive haemorrhage. The second phase is the preservation of future fertility, particularly since the prevalence of first-pregnancy ectopics is increasing. The first 8 to 10 weeks of a subsequent pregnancy are thus times of tension, and early ultrasound visualisation of intrauterine pregnancy is the best means of reassurance. In-vitro fertilisation offers the hope of a family for those in whom a second ectopic gestation has occurred and tubal anastomosis is not technically feasible.

Placental Abruption

The normally situated placenta undergoes many changes during pregnancy, so that its weight is several times greater than that of the foetus in the first trimester and reduces to 15%–20% of the weight of the newborn. During pregnancy areas of placental tissue cease to function, so that at term calcification and macroscopic areas of infarction are visible. Abnormal disruption of the uteroplacental junction produces retroplacental haemorrhage which, if small, results in a localised haematoma. Blood may track externally to the membranes, to pass through the cervix and become revealed bleeding. The amount of revealed bleeding will depend on the amount of haemorrhage and the proximity of the placenta to the cervical os. Blood may also track into the myometrium. The resulting syndrome will depend on the amount of placental disruption and the rate of extension, the amount of blood loss and the rate of loss and the degree of uterine myometrial destruction. Minor degrees of abruption will cause pain over a limited area of the uterus, which in turn will be irritable, contractile and tender to touch. The posterior placenta will not provide the same localising signs as a fundal or anterior placenta. Foetal disturbance and death will be related to the amount of placental disruption and its proximity to the cord insertion. The placenta has considerable reserve, but a small haematoma at the placental cord insertion may be sufficiently disruptive to produce foetal death. The classic acute abruptio placentae may be associated with trauma or more usually with hypertension, and relief of pain with morphine is mandatory. The real problem of diagnosis and management is to differentiate between spurious and premature labour in the minor cases. In the absence of revealed ante-partum loss an irritable contractile uterus should be considered abnormal. Relief of pain can be obtained with opiates, but subsequent monitoring necessitates hospital admission.

Gynaecological Problems and Pregnancy

Fibroids

Uterine fibromyomata in pregnancy increase in size in relation to myometrial hyperplasia. If they are more than 3–4 cm in diameter and are either subserous or pedunculated, then the diagnosis should have been made at the initial examination. If they are intramural a clinical diagnosis will suggest a discrepancy in uterine size rather than diagnosis of a fibroid. Larger fibroids should be noted without difficulty. The problems that give rise to pain will be due to torsion of the pedunculated fibroids or degeneration, which produces pain, tenderness and pyrexia. Cervical fibroids will cause pelvic discomfort by virtue of their size as well as pain in association with degeneration.

Fibroids are more common in women aged over 35, in multipara and in those who have a single pregnancy at an older age. The larger fibroids should be diagnosed clinically but diagnosis becomes more difficult as pregnancy progresses. Ultrasonography will provide the necessary supportive evidence for diagnosis. Pedunculated fibroids are rare, but torsion produces an acute episode of pain and a palpable tender swelling if it is not on the posterior surface of the uterus. Because of the tendency to conservatism in pregnancy, diagnostic delay is usual, and the necrosis induced by the pedicle torsion adds to the signs of degeneration.

Degeneration of subserous or intramural fibroid is more gradual, the pain being of low intensity and gradually becoming more persistent and severe. The site of tenderness will indicate the site of the fibroid. Because of the softening that occurs in pregnancy the contour of the fibroid will not be readily palpable. Uterine pain and tenderness, pyrexia and leucocytosis will depend on the size of the fibroid and degree of degeneration.

In the extreme case the fibroid will be almost cystic, and ultrasonography may not give a clear indication of its underlying structure. Differential diagnosis is difficult if the pain is severe and the fibroid cannot be outlined clinically or ultrasonographically. The guideline is that the signs are situated within the wall of the uterus. Appendicitis may produce adjacent uterine tenderness but not of the degree of fibromyomatas and degeneration.

The pedunculated fibroid that has undergone torsion will require laparotomy and excision. Other fibroids present and less pedunculated need not be removed.

The problem of degeneration is best managed by the relief of pain initially with pethidine or morphine and then other analgesics. Antibiotics are not necessary but will often have been started because of the pyrexia. The problem may recur but does not usually interfere with the outcome of labour. Pelvic fibroids may produce obstruction, and Caesarean section will be necessary. The smaller fibroids involute with the uterus in the post-partum phase and are unlikely to give rise to pain in the puerperium.

Ovarian Cysts

Ovarian or parovarian cysts are prone to torsion of the pedicle during the first half of pregnancy as the uterus rises out of the pelvis and immediately after delivery as the uterine size reduces rapidly. These shifts produce acute onset of pain. True cysts grow rapidly in the pregnant as in the non-pregnant state but do not give rise to pain unless torsion, pressure or intracystic haemorrhage occurs. Primary malignancy is less common in pregnant women with ovarian cysts because of their younger age.

The majority of small cysts are now diagnosed by routine ultrasound examination. The problem of cystic ovarian enlargement and true cyst formation has been discussed (see p. 73). The clinically palpable cyst is usually in the pouch of Douglas but can be anterior to the uterus in the case of dermoid cysts and will be confirmed by ultrasonography. The unilocular or multilocular anechoic appearance is diagnostic.

Because of the propensity to torsion, laparotomy and excision are necessary. The real problem arises if primary ovarian malignancy is detected.

Endometriosis

Pregnancy can occur in endometriosis. In the lesser degrees little peritoneal or ovarian tissue damage will have occurred, and the diagnosis may have been made laparoscopically during the investigation of infertility rather than pain. These lesser changes give rise to no distinct problems of pain in pregnancy, and the pregnancy may induce complete healing. In the severer degrees the endometriosis may have produced ovarian enlargement and peritoneal adhesion to the broad ligament, to the uterus or to the adjacent bowel. More rarely bowel or ureteric endometriosis will have produced minor degrees of stenosis which, with the advent of pregnancy, will give rise to partial obstructive symptoms. The main cause of pain will be the reduced mobility of the ovaries as the uterus grows. Ovarian endometriosis can result in leakage of inspissated blood with subsequent peritoneal irritation.

In patients with prepregnancy diagnosis of significant endometriosis the persistence of pain without palpable swelling or uterine tenderness will make differential diagnosis difficult. Sudden onset of pain in this group will bring about suspicion of rupture of an endometriotic cyst, but if there is no significant fresh bleeding the symptoms and signs will resolve within 48 to 72 hours. The tender nodulation of the pouch of Douglas characteristic of endometriosis is not present in pregnancy after the first trimester, the microscopic bleeding of endometriosis having been inhibited by pregnancy and tissue softening overcoming the fibrotic reaction. Occasionally diagnosis is made by chance at Caesarean section.

Endometriosis by definition resolves with pregnancy. The management problems arise not because of past bleeding but because of the fibrotic reaction that has occurred to such cyclic microscopic loss or to the accumulation of "chocolate blood" spilling into the peritoneal cavity which if severe will necessitate laparotomy.

4 Vulva, Vagina and Perineum

I. ROCKER and D. E. STURDY

Vulva and Vagina

I. Rocker

The vulva and vagina are involved by trauma, primary and secondary infections, dermatoses and neoplasia. Poor personal hygiene, chemical irritation and the spread of disease from the perineum and anus can all give rise to pain. The vulva is prone to be a site of irritation, which is in essence subliminal pain. In addition the vulval skin and vaginal mucosa are hormone sensitive and undergo the maturation changes of puberty, cyclical menstrual changes and atrophic changes after the menopause. The vulva is particularly sensitive to touch and pain, the vagina is less so, and the cervix is virtually insensitive. The possibility of direct inspection and examination of discharges and of tissues permits accurate diagnosis of pain. Conditions in which vaginal discharge is the predominant problem are more difficult to diagnose and resolve, in part because they are likely to be recurrent.

Trauma

Accidental trauma may occur during exercise, sport, bicycling and other transport injuries. Sexual trauma may be inadvertent or due to rape. Perineal and vaginal lacerations of delivery are common, and with early discharge from hospital need resolution once the mother is at home. Trauma from these various causes will be associated with varying degrees and persistence of pain and bleeding. The range extends, from a minor bruise to massive injuries involving the bladder, rectum and pelvic girdle.

The presence of bruising, haematoma formation and laceration of the vulva are readily obvious unless obscured by swelling. The swelling and tenderness may impede vaginal examination. The greater the external effects of trauma the more imperative is the need to exclude vaginal damage, so that examination under analgesia or anaesthesia should be undertaken. A small vulval bruise with continual vaginal bleeding should not be attributed to menstruation, since it may be due to vaginal vault laceration. Trauma due to an accident requires careful recording but trauma due to admitted or suspected sexual assault needs additional investigation. This should include taking specimens for sexually transmitted disease, for sperm detection and for genetic fingerprinting.

Once diagnosis has established the degree of trauma then the lesser problems will be resolved by giving analgesics and advice about reducing swelling of the vulva. Superficial lacerations may require suturing. With the advent of early post-delivery discharge from hospital, secondary suture of small perineal or vaginal or vulval lacerations discovered later, is not necessary.

A haematoma more than 5 cm in diameter requires drainage. The appearance of a vulval haematoma 24 hours after delivery is usually associated with a considerable lateral vaginal haematoma. Dependent evacuation will prevent the formation of an abscess, which could cause prolonged debility. Major trauma requires surgical correction, with particular attention to urethrovesical continuity and the prevention of urinary retention, which may proceed to retention with overflow.

Infections

Localised infections of the vulva and vagina are usually due to candida, trichomonas, chlamydia or herpes. Activation of commensal organisms can be associated with general ill-health, particularly when antibiotics have been used. The duration of menstrual loss, personal hygiene and habit are other significant factors. These infections are usually limited to the external genitalia but can spread to the internal pelvic organs. Whether papillomavirus, with or without visible warts, is always a transmitted infection and whether it is a primary infective agent, or becomes infective only in the presence of other predisposing conditions is unclear.

Acute infections may be so severe that antibiotic treatment is started before bacteriological investigations are begun. It cannot be emphasised enough that such practice is incorrect. The few moments it takes to collect the necessary swabs or blood sample from a severely ill patient would not be detrimental to treatment. The majority of vulvovaginal infections are low grade, and a significant number are recurrent. Thirty per cent are virtually asymptomatic and are only discovered during the course of routine cytology or other examination. Many patients have combined infections.

Herpes ulceration is very painful and may be difficult to differentiate from candidal ulcers unless the vesicular stage of herpes is seen. Vulval or vaginal warts are readily seen, and care should be taken with local treatment, particularly with podophyllin, not to produce unnecessary ulceration. Severe candidosis with its caseous plaques and curdy discharge is relatively rare, the majority of candida infections being difficult to differentiate from

Trichomonas vaginalis infection, particularly if there is secondary infection with *Gardenerella* or other bacteria.

Chronic or recurrent pain associated with vulvovaginal infections may be attributed in part to anxiety arising from the patient's understandable reluctance to discuss the possibility of sexually transmitted disease.

Bartholin's Cyst and Abscess

Blockage of the duct of Bartholin's gland causes distension of the duct to form a cyst (Fig. 4.1). Infection with *Escherichia coli* or other vulval or vaginal pathogens will produce an abscess with oedema of the overlying labium majus and arises within 3 to 5 days of the occlusion. The swelling can be confused with an abscess arising from a hair follical or sebaceous gland.

Bartholin's abscess is visible as a reddened tender swelling, in most cases unilateral, in the lower half of the labium majus. There is moderate to severe pain with malaise and pyrexia. If untreated the abscess will usually rupture into the vagina, the perineum or externally. Fluctuation indicates the need for urgent treatment to prevent this.

Antibiotics alone will not resolve the problem unless there is spontaneous recannulisation of the duct. If rupture is imminent, marsupialisation offers a chance of a pseudoduct being maintained and preventing recurrence. However, the size of the abscess may mean that simple incision and dependent drainage will be the emergency treatment. Recurrence of the condition may best be resolved by awaiting a quiescent phase and excising the pseudocyst and Bartholin's gland. The latter is not readily demarcated, so there is always a chance of failure. In addition, vascularity of the labium

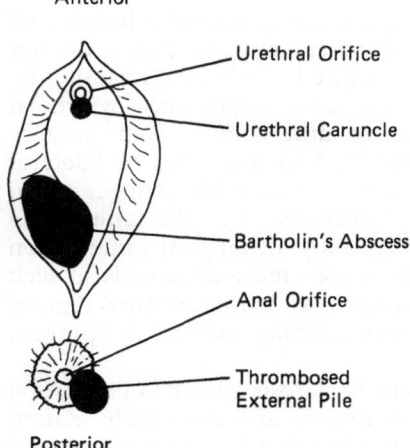

Fig. 4.1. The vulva and perineum: sites of urethral caruncle, Bartholin's abscess and thrombosed external pile.

is such that there is a considerable risk of postoperative haematoma formation, which may take several weeks to clear.

Vulval Tumours

Benign tumours are of epidermal or sebaceous origin, rarely painful and not clinically distinctive. Removal is cosmetic or because of recurrent infection. A rare problem is a profusion of sebaceous glands, which will cause discomfort because of the associated vulval enlargement, which may require partial vulvectomy. Benign pigmented naevi occur and can undergo malignant change. Lipomas, fibromas and neurofibromas are best excised, particularly if pedunculated.

The changing pattern of nomenclature of vulval dystrophy does not remove the need for the careful assessment of a single ulcer which persists or grows, or of a non-healing fissure. Both types of lesion are usually painful and if secondarily infected may heal, only to recur at the same site within 2 to 4 weeks. Excision biopsy is necessary, though preliminary cytology can be helpful.

Laser treatment of vulval carcinoma-in-situ is effective and, unlike vulvectomy, does not cause disfigurement. Frank malignancy is usually due to squamous carcinoma of the vulva, which presents as a growing ulcer to an extensive exophytic mass. Basal cell carcinoma is less common but amenable to a more limited excision. Melanoma of the vulva also occurs and requires specialist treatment.

Vulval Dystrophy/Dermatoses

The vulva is prone to eczematous, allergic and rarely psoriatic lesions, all liable to secondary infection and constant irritation. Usually there are other skin lesions, and a dermatologist's help is required. Chronic irritation by contact or scratching will produce a leukoplakic appearance which, if secondarily infected, becomes impossible to differentiate from primary leukoplakia. In the younger woman it can lead to unilateral or bilateral vulval hypertrophy and in the older woman with atrophic changes to an appearance very similar to leukoplakia or lichen sclerosis, the latter being more prone to fissuring and ulceration, which only histological examination can differentiate. Malignant transformation is seen more commonly in such skin changes, which therefore require careful and continued surveillance. Preventive vulvectomy is disfiguring and disheartening and will not prevent the recurrence of lichen sclerosis.

The management of leukoplakia and lichen sclerosis consists of attention to personal hygiene and avoidance of all allergic and chemically irritant materials. A light covering at night and a loose crotch clothing both day and night is helpful. Application of 1% hydrocortisone lotion at night will reduce itching and so scratching. It is often difficult to establish whether the loss of sleep is due to the irritation or whether poor sleep habit is aggravating the sensation of itching.

Postmenopausal periurethral and inner labial atrophy, originally designated kraurosis vulvae, is readily recognised because of its punctate ecchymoses, almost purple in patches, and contraction of the introitus. Coitus becomes painful because of the contraction and the fissuring that occurs. Treatment of secondary infection and hormone replacement therapy are indicated. Unfortunately the majority of patients present in their sixties, by which age the contraction may be too great to be overcome.

Vaginal Tumours

Cysts of varying size that occur in the wall of the vagina are commonly the vestigial remains of the Wolffian duct. They rarely need removal, and their proximity to the bladder or continuity into the broad ligament can make surgery difficult. Vaginal adenosis can occur in peri and post pubertal women whose mothers were given diethylstilboestrol during pregnancy. Diagnosis is by cytology and histology. The peak of such usage was in the early 1960s, and individuals exposed to the hormone in utero are now under regular cytological follow-up.

Malignancy is usually due to spread from cervical cancer. Suburethral secondaries from endometrial carcinoma also occur. Differentiation between primary and secondary vaginal cancer can be impossible and surgical treatment is effective only if sufficient lateral tissue clearance can be obtained. Vaginectomy is total.

Vaginal Cervix

The vaginal cervix, though relatively insensitive, is associated with considerable morbidity both due to direct contact pain and pain spreading to the lower abdomen, the groins and low back. Unfortunately, cervicitis has become a blanket name which should preferably be restricted to true infection of the cervix. Under hormonal influence the squamous epithelium of the ectocervix and the epithelium of the squamocolumnar junction undergo cyclical changes. Desquamation of the squamous epithelium by coitus, pregnancy and labour allows the more vascular columnar epithelium to extend over the ectocervix. In many young women the squamocolumnar junction is readily visible and its appearance is enhanced by use of the contraceptive pill. Traumatic eversion of the cervix in labour produces an open patulous os, which permits direct contact of the columnar lining of the endocervix. This surface is more prone to infection and so produces a reaction which will depend on whether it is limited to the cervix (cervicitis) or whether it spreads to the parametrium (parametritis) or to the base of the bladder ("trigonitis"). Excessive discharge and postcoital bleeding may occur. A lesion revealed on routine inspection of a symptomfree woman's cervix should not be termed a cervical ulcer unless this is really the case. If symptomatic, the term cervical erosion or desquamation can safely be used, and the patient should be told that the surface of the cervix is grazed and that cauterisation will produce a firmer fibrotic surface. An enlarged cervix with immobility due to parametrial fibrosis will in most cases require hysterectomy.

Cervical Intraepithelial Neoplasia

This is not itself associated with pain, but the abnormality is more common in women who have other predisposing factors to vaginal and pelvic infection. Successful treatment of the cervical changes will not necessarily relieve any associated pain.

Perineum

D.E. Sturdy

Acute Painful Conditions of the Perineum

Thrombosed External Pile (Perianal Haematoma)

A thrombosed external pile (a haematoma formed on rupture of a vein at the anal verge) occurs most commonly in horseriders and yachtsmen or after a long car journey on hard seating. Thrombosed external piles can be recurrent.

The haematoma appears as a rapidly forming dark plum coloured swelling at the anal verge (Fig. 4.1). It is very tender on digital pressure and the patient will resist rectal examination because of the tenderness.

A thrombosed external pile will resolve in 7 to 10 days. In the acute phase (the first 48 hours) incision and evacuation of the haematoma under local anaesthesia will relieve the pain.

Acute Fissure in Ano

A fissure in the lining of the lower end of the anal canal below the pectinate line (Fig. 4.2) is initiated by the passage of hard constipated stools. Fifty per cent of acute fissures become chronic.

Acute fissure in ano is characterised by sudden onset of severe pain aggravated by defaecation and persisting for 2 to 3 hours after going to stool. Defaecation is followed by pruritus and frequent light pink-coloured bleeding. On examination a split can be seen at the anal verge, usually midline and posterior, which is extremely tender on palpation. A sentinel pile is evident at the posterior end of the fissure (Fig. 4.2). The patient will resist rectal examination, which is very painful.

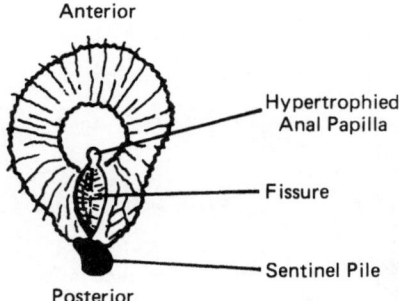

Fig. 4.2. Fissure in ano.

Acute fissure in ano is managed by elimination of constipation with suppositories and mild aperients with application of a local anaesthetic ointment (Anithaine) after passage of stool. If the condition does not respond within 6 weeks the patient should be admitted for an anal stretch procedure (Lords) under general anaesthesia.

Prolapsed Internal Piles

Internal haemorrhoids per se are painless, but large third-degree piles may prolapse through the anal orifice, where they may swell alarmingly, owing to spasm of the anal sphincteric muscles. Prolapsing piles may be associated with a rectal tumour.

Prolapsed internal piles are characterised by continuous pain, discharge and bleeding in the anal region. Classically three plum coloured pile masses will be seen protruding outside the anal orifice, and there will be surrounding oedema and bloody mucoid discharge. Rectal examination may not be possible.

Hot baths, local ice packs, and local anaesthetic ointments will reduce the pile masses within 2 to 3 weeks. Haemorrhoidectomy is recommended if there is no improvement within 3 months. When the acute phase has passed the large bowel should be examined thoroughly with sigmoidoscopy and a barium enema to exclude colorectal disease.

Perianal Abscess

A perianal abscess arises in the subcutaneous tissues at the anal margin as a result of infection in an anal gland, a hair follicle, a sweat gland, a perianal haematoma or an anal fissure. An untreated abscess will rupture, most commonly to the exterior on the anal skin or, less frequently, internally into the anal canal.

On examination the painful, throbbing, tender abscess will be seen as a swelling (frequently fluctuant) at the anal verge (Fig. 4.3). Examination of the rectum will be painful for the patient and should be avoided.

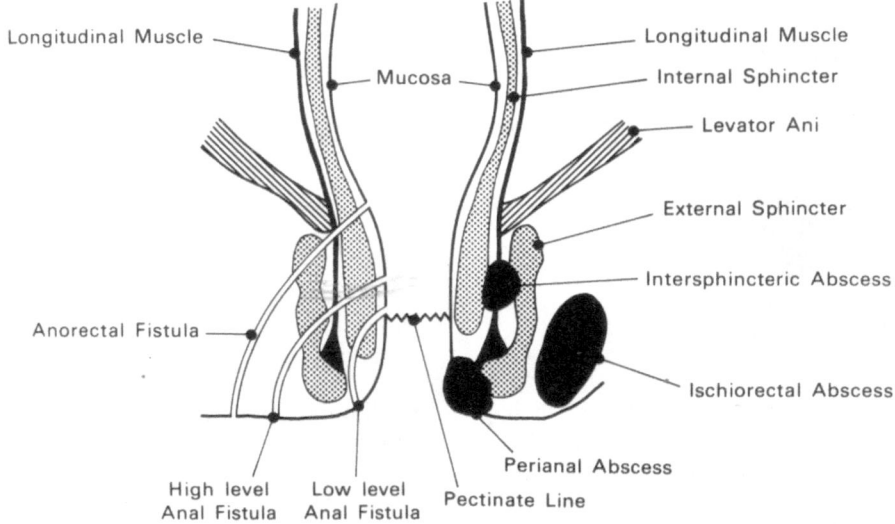

Fig. 4.3. Sites of anorectal fistulae and abscesses.

A perianal abscess should be managed with incision and drainage to the exterior and frequent hot baths.

Ischiorectal Abscess

An ischiorectal abscess is caused by *Escherichia coli* infection of the lax areolar tissue of the ischiorectal fossa. The majority of such infections are blood borne. An abscess may follow instrumental injury to the rectum or inflamed haemorrhoids and their surgical treatment. The forming abscess bulges medially into the rectum and anal canal and inferiorly into the perineum. Palpable softening of the abscess wall leads to rupture into the rectum and anal canal or more rarely into the perineum. Fifty per cent of ischiorectal abscesses result in anal fistulae: 5 % are associated with Crohn's disease or ulcerative colitis.

Diagnosis is both by visual inspection and palpation. Examination will reveal a tender indurated swelling bulging into the perineum with redness and oedema of overlying skin. The constitutional effects are malaise and pyrexia. Throbbing pain of the affected perineum and buttock will be aggravated by sitting and defaecation. A rectal examination is essential to palpate the bulging tender mass in the lateral rectal wall.

Ischiorectal abscess is managed with early external incision and drainage of the abscess, light packing of the cavity, and frequent hot baths.

Chronic Painful Conditions of the Perineum

Chronic Fissure in Ano

Fifty per cent of acute anal fissures become chronic. The edges of the fissure become indurated, and the circular fibres of the internal sphincter muscle may be exposed in the base of the fissure. At the lower end a cutaneous, tender, infected and oedematous "sentinel tag" may form (Fig. 4.2). Five per cent of chronic fissures are associated with Crohn's disease of the bowel.

The patient will have a history of a previous acute fissure of 3 months' or more duration and occasional acute exacerbations with bleeding. The presence of a "sentinel tag" externally, oedematous anal papilla internally (Fig. 4.2) and tenderness on digital examination complete the diagnosis.

Chronic fissures are usually managed by daily anal stretching with a dilator. Anal stretch procedures under general anaesthesia will cure less than 20 % of chronic anal fissures. Chronic fissures can also be treated surgically by fissurectomy and sphincterotomy (division of the lower part of the internal sphincter muscle either through the base of the excised fissure or by a separate lateral incision).

All patients with a chronic anal fissure should be examined endoscopically and radiologically for evidence of chronic inflammatory disease of the large bowel.

Fistula in Ano

A fistula in ano is an epithelialised tract connecting the anal canal to the skin. The majority of fistulae are an end result of an ischiorectal abscess (p. 88). Multiple or persistent fistulae may occur in Crohn's disease (5 % to 8 %) or more rarely in ulcerative colitis (2 % to 3 %). Anal fistulae are either high or low (Fig. 4.3). Low level fistulae enter the anal canal at or below the pectinate line and traverse the distal part of the internal sphincter. High level fistulae open internally above the pectinate line and may traverse through both internal and external sphincter muscles.

Patients with anal fistulae have a history of anorectal abscesses with chronic perineal and perianal discomfort and a purulent, often bloody, discharge. The fistulous opening discharges pus on digital pressure into the anal canal. Digital and endoscopic examination may identify the internal opening of the fistula.

Management of anal fistulae consists of laying open the fistulous tract to allow free drainage. Great care is needed to avoid damage to the anorectal muscular ring. Biopsies of the fistulous tract are required to exclude Crohn's disease or ulcerative colitis.

Rectal Prolapse

Prolapse of the rectum through the anal orifice may occur in infancy or in the latter decades of life. Rectal prolapse causes pelvic pain and discomfort.

Infantile rectal prolapse is a self-limiting condition resulting from inadequate bowel training and straining at stool. Ten percent of young children affected will have an associated pedunculated (juvenile) polyp, which may bleed briskly when constricted by the sphincter muscle. The prolapse is managed by restoration of normal bowel habit and the polyp by ligation and excision.

An *adult rectal prolapse* is a sliding hernia which involves first the anterior and later the posterior rectal wall. It is commoner in elderly patients and is the result of poor sphincteric control. Contributory factors are obesity, chronic bronchitis, haemorrhoids and a history of difficult parturition. The prolapse gives rise to dragging pain in the perineum and on examination can be seen as a dark red swelling protruding through the anal orifice. The exposed rectal mucosa bleeds, produces mucus in large quantities and may ulcerate. The swelling is easily reducible through the patulous anal orifice but reappears immediately on coughing or straining. Disease of the terminal large bowel, which may produce a prolapse of the rectum, must be excluded by endoscopy and barium studies (which, however, may be difficult because of laxity of the anal musculature). Prolapse in the very elderly and minor degrees of prolapse may be controlled by the insertion of a subcutaneous circumanal wire structure (Thiersch operation). Larger prolapses will need surgical repair. Repair from below is by a muscle buttress procedure. Repair from above is either by insertion of Ivalon sponge into the presacral space or by anterior resection of the rectum. All operative procedures carry a 30 % recurrence rate.

Carcinoma of the Anal Canal

The upper half (2.5 cm) of the anal canal has columnar epithelium, and a carcinoma in that area will be an adenocarcinoma. Malignant tumours arising in the lower half of the anal canal (which has squamous epithelium) will be squamous cell carcinomas. Adenocarcinoma spreads locally and to pararectal and internal iliac nodes. Squamous cell carcinoma spreads locally and to the inguinal lymph nodes. Other malignant tumours of the anal canal are basal-cell carcinomas and melanomas.

A carcinoma in the anal canal causes constant anal discomfort, pain on defaecation, persistent and offensive bloody discharge and a constant feeling of something causing pressure in the canal. Digital examination reveals a hard-edged ulcer, which leaves blood on the examining finger. Both inguinal regions should be examined for lymphadenopathy. Anoscopy, biopsy for histological confirmation of malignancy and sigmoidoscopy to exclude disease of the rectum and sigmoid colon are mandatory.

The majority of patients need abdominoperineal excision of the rectum with wide excision of the perianal skin. Inguinal block dissection will be necessary if inguinal lymph nodes are involved. Elderly and frail patients should be treated with interstitial radium needles or external radiotherapy.

Perineal Recurrence after Treatment of Pelvirectal Tumours

Tumours may recur in the pelvis and perineum after an abdominoperineal or anterior resection of the rectum or after a Hartmann procedure. Pelvic recurrence is particularly liable to occur where the original operation has been only palliative or where malignant tissue has been left in the presacral space. Perineal recurrence may also be found in patients after palliative local or external radiotherapy treatment for irresectable malignant tumours of the rectum or genital tract. Involvement of somatic sacral and perineal nerves produces intractable pain in these patients.

Perineal recurrence will appear as a hard indurated mass in the perineum, with evidence, on vaginal examination, of fixation to the walls of the pelvic cavity and possibly involvement of the upper vagina. The diagnosis is confirmed by percutaneous or pervaginal biopsy.

Treatment can only be palliative. External radiotherapy may benefit some patients, but chemotherapy has little to offer. For patients with intractable pain due to involvement of somatic pelvic or perineal nerves, a nerve block with alcohol or phenol may be helpful (see Chapter 8).

5 Bladder and Renal Tract

D. E. STURDY

Pain in the Anterior (Urinary) Compartment of the Female Pelvis

The autonomic nerve supply to the urinary bladder and urethra consists of sympathetic fibres from cord segments T12 and L1, 2 and 3 parasympathetic fibres and S2, 3 and 4 (Fig. 1.3). Pain sensation and discomfort in the bladder, transmitted centrally by these autonomic nerves, can be initiated by inflammation, spasm or distension or by obstruction to the bladder outlet. Pain in the bladder may be acute or chronic. Acute pain can arise from cystourethritis and retention of urine, and chronic pain from cystitis, retention, bladder irritability, bladder calculi and advanced carcinoma of the bladder. Bladder pain, both acute and chronic, may be initiated by a combination of infection, spasm and obstruction. The female patient is very prone to bladder infections, and bladder symptoms are not uncommonly present when the primary disorder is located in the gynaecological or intestinal compartment of the pelvis.

Pain in the intrapelvic ureter is initiated by obstruction, which may be within the ureter or in the wall of the ureter. Ureteric pain is due to spasm and contraction of the muscular wall of the ureter and is transmitted centrally by autonomic fibres from the sympathetic (T11, 12; L1, 2, 3) and parasympathetic (S2, 3, 4) plexuses (Fig. 1.3). Ureteric pain may be acute or chronic, acute pain being caused by obstruction due to a calculus and chronic pain by calculus, obstruction, stricture, tumour or external compression.

Urethral Caruncle

A uretheral caruncle is a granulomatous tumour sited at the margin of the external urethral orifice (Fig. 4.1). The aetiology of the tumour, which occurs mostly in elderly women, is unknown. A caruncle does not always produce symptoms but can cause frequency of micturition, terminal discomfort, and pain on touch and dyspareunia. It does not usually bleed.

Urethral caruncle is diagnosed by visual inspection. It must be differentiated from a primary urethral neoplasm, which, however, is very rare.

A caruncle, if producing symptoms, can be treated with coagulation diathermy.

Acute Bladder Pain

Acute Cystourethritis

Acute bacterial cystitis is very common in women, most of whom will have at least one attack during their lifetime. The proximity of the urethral orifice to the vagina accounts for ascending infection in many patients and is undoubtedly the route of infection in the catheterised bladder. The bladder can also become infected from the bloodstream or by descending infection from the kidneys. The symptoms of acute bladder inflammation are frequency, urgency, pain on micturition, suprapubic discomfort, fever and occasionally haematuria, with tenderness over the bladder on suprapubic compression. Details of laboratory diagnosis and management are discussed in Chapter 2.

Acute Retention of Urine

The obstructed distended bladder is acutely painful and is palpable as a tender midline mass arising out of the pelvis in the hypogastric region. Acute retention sometimes follows instrumentation or catheterisation of the bladder in operative procedures in the lower abdomen and pelvis. All other cases are due to bacterial infection of the bladder, neck and urethra, or to swellings in the pelvis.

Urgent catheterisation is needed to empty the bladder and relieve pain. Systemic antibiotic cover should be given for the period the urethral catheter is in situ.

Chronic Bladder Pain

Chronic Retention of Urine

The chronically obstructed bladder is relatively painless, the patient usually complaining of lower abdominal discomfort and an increase in abdominal girth. The bladder is easily palpable in the hypogastrium, arising out of the pelvis and dull to percussion. Differential diagnosis is between an enlarged or gravid uterus and an ovarian cyst. The obstructed bladder develops saccules and diverticulae, which in many cases become secondarily infected.

The infection may lead to the formation of bladder stones. The commonest cause of chronic retention of urine is a neurogenic outlet obstruction or (more rarely) a bladder outlet stenosis. Advanced tumours of the cervix may rarely produce chronic urinary retention. Diagnosis is established by a pelvic ultrasound scan. Catheterisation will decompress the bladder but should only be undertaken with full sterile precautions to avoid introducing infection into the obstructed lower urinary tract.

Chronic Cystitis (Chronic Interstitial Cystitis)

The chronically infected bladder is usually contracted and not palpable and may be the result of repeated acute infection. In a few middle-aged women an autoimmune reaction may be an aetiological factor, and at cystoscopy an "ulcer" may be seen in the vault of the bladder (Hunner's ulcer). The patient complains of frequent, urgent micturition but passes small volumes of urine. Haematuria and hypogastric discomfort are also present. The urine is sterile.

Overdistending the bladder under anaesthesia (hydrostatic distension) may be helpful. Intractable cases may need enlargement of bladder capacity with a loop of ileum or caecum, or total cystectomy and an ileal loop conduit.

Schistosomiasis of the Bladder

This condition, endemic in Egypt, East Africa and the Far East, is due to infestation of the bladder with the adult worm of *Schistosoma haematobium*. The ova, excreted into the bladder, cause fibrosis, producing a small contracted bladder. Squamous cell metaphasia and invasive carcinoma occur in 30 % of cases. The bladder infestation produces chronic pain in the anterior compartment of the pelvis and haematuria. Treatment is with praziquantel, oxamniquine or metriphonate. Schistosomiasis, previously rare in the United Kingdom, is seen more often these days due to immigration of people from infected areas.

Tuberculosis of the Bladder

In a proportion of tuberculosis patients the infection involves the bladder, which becomes small and contracted (Fig. 5.1). The patient experiences extreme frequency and urgency of micturition with haematuria. The bladder lesions of tuberculosis are a manifestation of systemic and genitourinary tuberculosis, and treatment is with antituberculous therapy for 18 months to 2 years, combined with procedures for enlargement of bladder capacity if the disease is intractable.

Bladder Calculi

Bladder calculi are rare in Western society but are more frequently encountered in women of Turkish, Middle Eastern and Far Eastern origin.

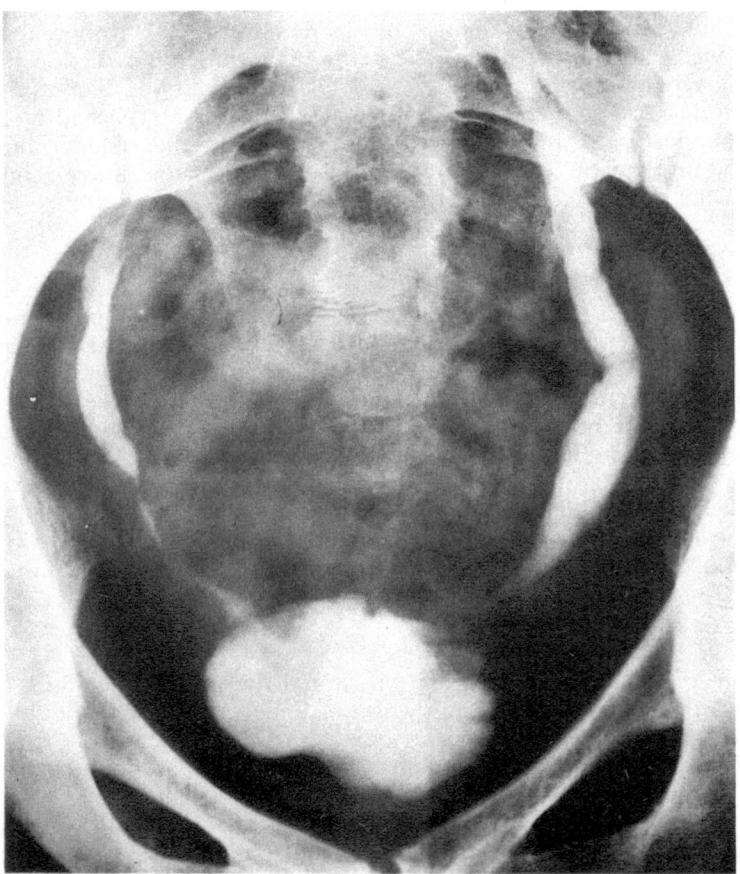

Fig. 5.1. Small contracted bladder with hydroureters demonstrated by IVU.

The calculi form in obstructed and infected bladders, around foreign bodies in the bladder or as a result of enlargement of ureteric stones which have passed into the bladder. Stones within the bladder are associated with recurrent attacks of urinary infection, bladder discomfort and sometimes haematuria (Fig. 5.2). A characteristic symptom of a bladder stone is interruption of micturition when the calculus becomes impacted in the internal urinary meatus in midstream and abruptly shuts off the urinary flow, causing an acute pain in the urethra and bladder. The stones should be crushed and removed endoscopically. Corrective surgery to the bladder outlet may be necessary if outlet obstruction is an aetiological factor in producing the stones.

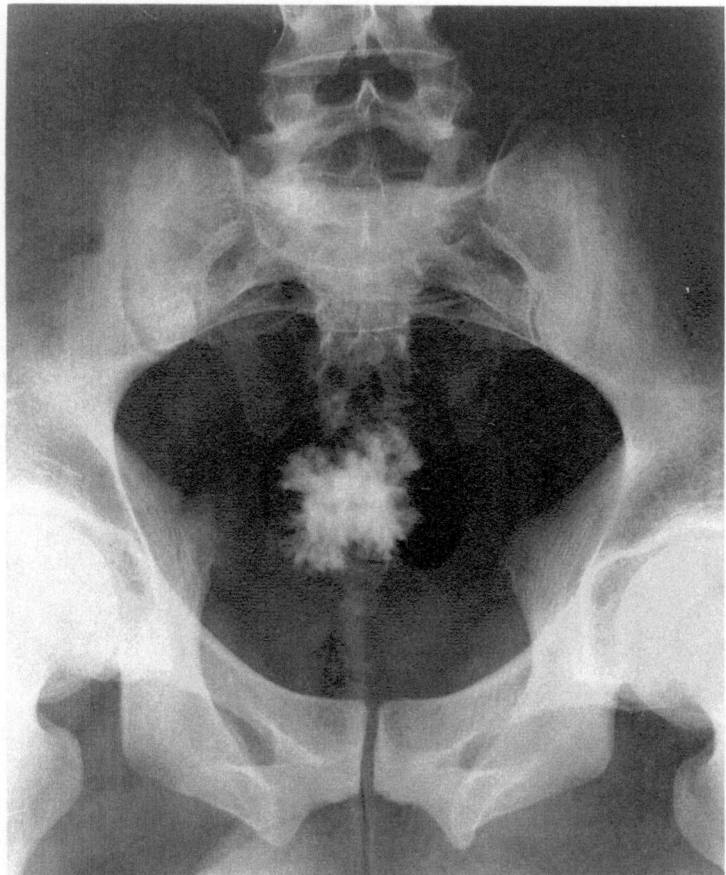

Fig. 5.2. Pelvic x-ray showing a spiculated bladder calculus.

The Unstable Bladder

In this condition, characteristically confined to neurotic middle-aged women, the patient has an uncontrollable desire to empty the bladder when it is only partially full (under 250 ml). Micturition proceeds normally, but the patient may experience urge incontinence and bladder discomfort owing to excessive contractions of the bladder detrusor muscles. The cause of precipitate micturition is failure of higher centres to exert their inhibitory effect on the sacral parasympathetic plexuses. Instability of the bladder is easily demonstrated by urodynamic studies. Surgery has no place in the management of bladder instability. Drugs that inhibit bladder contractility may be beneficial. Those in common use are imipramine hydrochloride and propantheline bromide.

Pain from Advanced Carcinoma of the Bladder

Bladder tumours are not painful in the early stages. The commonest presenting symptom in 90 % of T1, T2 bladder cancers is painless haematuria. Advanced tumours (T3 and T4) will have infiltrated outside the bladder wall and become adherent to the symphysis anteriorly, the cervix and uterus posteriorly and the lateral pelvic wall (Fig. 5.3). Infiltration of the surrounding organs produces visceral pelvic pain, whilst involvement of the lateral walls of the pelvis produces somatic pain. Infiltration of the bladder wall itself leads to visceral pain and bleeding, often accompanied by secondary infection, and the enlarging tumour may obstruct one or both ureters. Death from an untreated or recurrent carcinoma of the bladder with strangury, severe pain and bleeding is one of the most miserable deaths known to man. Treatment of advanced bladder carcinomas can at best be only palliative. Radiotherapy may be beneficial in some patients. A palliative cystectomy is sometimes the only treatment that can be offered.

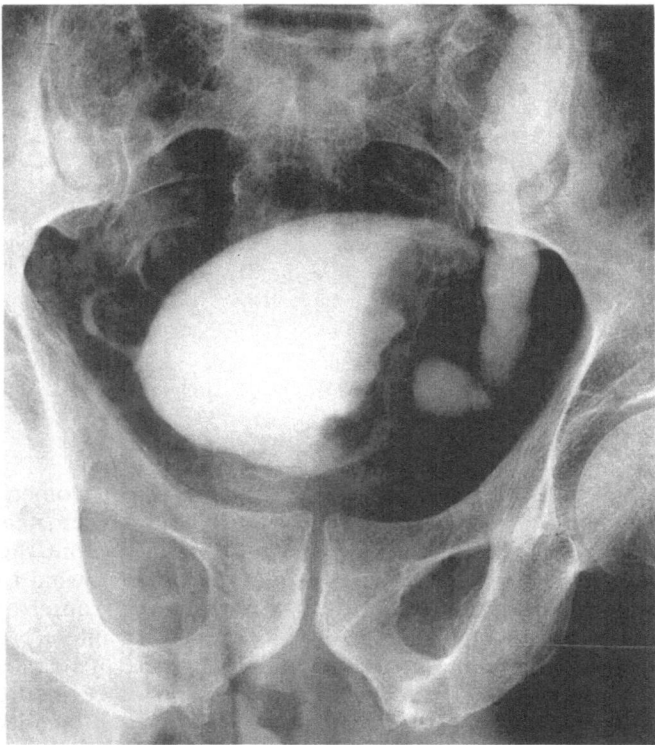

Fig. 5.3. Bladder carcinoma with left ureteric obstruction (IVU).

Pain in the Intrapelvic Ureter

Pain in the intrapelvic segment of the ureter is initiated by obstruction, which either may be in the wall of the ureter or may be due to a calculus within the ureter.

Acute pain can be caused by:

Impacted stone (ureteric colic)
Rarely a clot in the ureter (clot colic).

Chronic pain can be caused by:

Longstanding stone impaction
Stricture of ureter (after stone impaction, after surgery, in tuberculosis or schistomiasis)
Obstruction by a bladder neoplasm
Obstruction by a tumour of another pelvic organ

Acute Ureteric Pain

Ureteric Colic

The acute pain of an obstructed ureter is produced by spasm of the ureter behind the obstructing lesion, in the greater majority of cases an impacted calculus. All ureteric calculi have their origin in the kidney, and about 60 % will pass into the bladder without surgical interference. Obstruction to the flow of urine down the ureter compromises excretion from the kidney and may lead to diminution or cessation of excretion from the affected side. A near-complete ureteric obstruction with a sterile urine can be safely treated conservatively for up to 8 weeks in the knowledge that complete recovery of renal function will occur when the obstruction is relieved. Rapid deterioration in renal function will occur when urine, under pressure in an obstructed urinary tract, is infected. In this situation urgent surgical intervention is essential.

Ureteric colic produces the severest pain known to man. Classically the pain starts in the costovertebral angle and, as the stone passes distally, becomes evident in the groin, genitalia and sometimes the front of the thigh. The pain is intense and colicky and may last several hours. The patient will be in shock and vomiting and 40 % of patients have frank haematuria due to damage to the ureteric urothelium. The rest will have microscopic haematuria. Clinical examination will reveal a shocked patient with tenderness in the costovertebral angle and, in many cases, tenderness and guarding in the iliac fossa. Pyrexia is an ominous sign and may indicate infection behind an impacted stone. Eighty-five per cent of urinary calculi contain some calcium and are radio-opaque. A plain X-ray film of the pelvis may demonstrate a calculus along the line of the ureter within the pelvis (Fig.

5.4). An intravenous urogram during the bout of ureteric colic (an essential investigation) demonstrates delayed excretion in the kidney on the affected side (nephrogenic phase) and may show the site of impaction of the calculus in delayed films taken 2 to 3 hours after administration of the contrast medium. Only rarely is retrograde ureterography necessary to demonstrate the site of impaction of the stone.

A patient with ureteric colic needs urgent hospital admission and administration of large doses of analgesics, such as pethidine or morphine and atropine, and a liberal fluid intake. Provided the patient is apyrexial and the urine sterile an expectant policy may be adopted, for 6 to 8 weeks if necessary, because stones of less than 5 mm in diameter may be expected to pass spontaneously. During this observation period weekly KUB (kidneys, ureter, bladder) films are taken to assess distal progression of the stone.

In pyrexial patients with acute loin pain and tenderness and evidence of bacterial infection in the urine, urgent kidney drainage by nephrostomy is undertaken, and systemic antibiotics are administered. Stones larger than 5 mm in diameter may need to be removed surgically. Retrograde retrieval with wire baskets (Dormia) or direct removal by ureteroscopy will successfully recover the majority of calculi. Ureteroscopy is easier in the female than the male, and the percentage of stones recovered is consequently higher in the female. Larger calculi can be disintegrated by ultrasound under direct vision at ureteroscopy. Recovery of calculi in the pelvic segment of the ureter is possible in 95 % of patients, using the above techniques. Lithotripsy (external disintegration by high-frequency ultrasound waves) has little application in the management of stones in the distal ureter. Ureterolithotomy (open operative removal of a stone in the ureter) is necessary in under 5 % of patients with stones in the pelvic ureter.

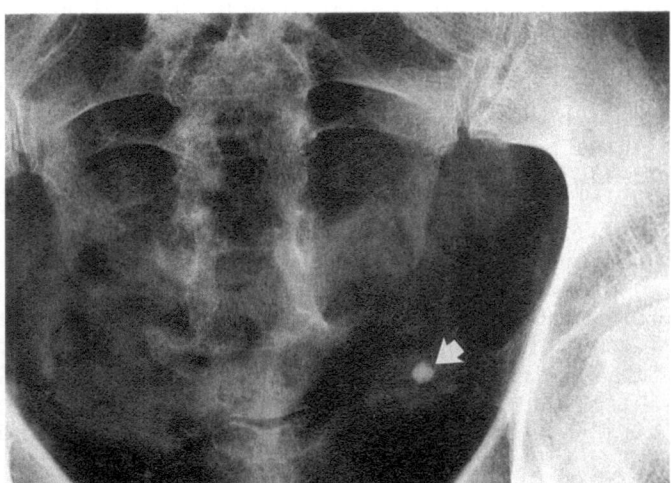

Fig. 5.4. Straight radiograph showing a left ureteric calculus.

Chronic Ureteric Pain

In the absence of complete ureteric obstruction a calculus may remain impacted in the pelvic ureter for months or years and will usually increase in size during this period. The patient may experience infrequent attacks of mild ureteric colic, but the principal symptom is chronic pain in the iliac fossa, which must be distinguished from the discomfort of diverticular or appendicular disease, chronic salpingitis and pelvic endometriosis. In rare instances a large calculus impacted in the left ureterovesical junction may be palpable in the vaginal fornix. With the exception of symptomless stones in the very elderly patient, most of these calculi will need to be removed by the surgical procedures outlined above. The pelvic ureter may also be chronically obstructed by a stricture following stone impaction, by tumours of the cervix, uterus, ovaries and rectum and by bladder tumours involving the ureteric orifice. The chronic ureteric pain produced by these disorders is overshadowed by pain from the primary disease in the pelvic cavity or bladder, and the surgeon's aim in the management of these patients will be eradication of the primary disease and reimplantation of the obstructed ureter into the bladder.

In the rare instance where the pelvic or vesical disease involves both ureters, a urinary diversionary procedure is necessary and an ileal loop conduit can be created for relief of pain and chronic ureteric obstruction.

6 Gynaecological Pain

I. ROCKER

Uterovaginal Prolapse

Uterovaginal prolapse can cause low-grade and persistent pain. Vaginal prolapse can occur without uterine descent, the stretched anterior wall persisting as a cystocele or a urethro-cystocele. Vault prolapse with uterine descent will be present if the paracervical tissues have been damaged or overstretched and if the peritoneal pouch of Douglas is anatomically deep. Deficiencies of the perineum and the adjacent levator muscle produce rectoceles. The short deficient perineum allows the descending cystocele and the cervix to be readily visible and to touch the labia, producing the sensation of a lump. The cystocele contains the bladder, and urinary frequency with or without stress incontinence is common. Similarly the levator defect may cause ineffective emptying of the rectum. Uterovaginal prolapse is therefore a combination of basic anatomical structure, the effects of pregnancy and labour, postmenopausal hormone deficiency and poor general muscular fitness. The addition of obesity, chronic cough and constipation makes permanent correction difficult. Secondary prolapse may occur with large intrapelvic tumours or following surgical resection, such as abdominoperineal rectal excision or total vulvectomy. Pain is primarily due to stretching of the ligamentous supports and secondarily to the excoriation that can occur to the prolapsed cervical or vaginal tissue. A minor degree of prolapse can be associated with retroversion of the uterus, which in itself can produce pressure on the rectum or transmitted dyspareunia if an ovary is prolapsing into the dependent pouch of Douglas. The pattern of prolapse has altered with changing obstetric practice, fewer pregnancies, shorter duration of labour and non-traumatic forceps deliveries. The progression of prolapse varies but when of increasing severity the changes are usually apparent within one to two years.

Fear of prolapse is well founded. In past decades the majority of problems have been associated with procidentia, and understandably the fear has been the progression of a prolapse to this severity. Procidentia occurs in only about 10 % of prolapses, and it is this form which can be associated with major urinary problems, occasionally poor faecal control and eventual decubitus ulceration and limited mobility. The indignities suffered by women of the not too distant past are still known to the present generation. The most common error is to label as prolapse the natural descent of the anterior vaginal wall or cervical descent by traction with an attached tenaculum. The latter will most commonly take place at postnatal examination or during routine examinations, e.g. for cervical cytology or contraception. The comment that a prolapse exists when a woman is free of symptoms should be very carefully considered in order not to cause anxiety. Minor degrees of prolapse do not respond significantly to reconstructive surgery. In the investigation of backache other causes should be sought before the pain is attributed to prolapse. The pain of prolapse is central, suprapubic and dragging in the groins and is relieved by rest. There is a sensation of a lump at the vulva, which is also relieved by lying down but may be aggravated by sitting, walking, coughing or straining. There are no significant abdominal physical signs.

Diagnosis is best made visually, with the patient in the lithotomy or left lateral or Sims' position. The use of a Sims' speculum will allow assessment of the cystocele and of cervical descent. The pressure of the speculum on the posterior wall will enable the examiner to avoid the error of misdiagnosing an enterocele as a cystocele. Combined rectovaginal examination resolves any difficulty in assessing the degree of rectocele.

The younger active woman with a second degree prolapse (i.e. in which the cervix descends to the vulva) will be best served by vaginal hysterectomy and repair. Occasionally such change is seen in a woman aged 25 to 30 after the birth of her first child, and in such a case repair is best postponed until childbearing is complete. The older woman will benefit from either vaginal hysterectomy or a Manchester repair, and the decision is best made at the time of operation. Surgical correction of prolapse for elderly women confined to bed or a wheelchair seems unwarranted, in spite of requests from relatives: unfortunately surgery in such patients cannot guarantee urinary continence.

The postoperative sequelae of pelvic floor surgery are a considerable problem. The immediate ones are related to vaginal discharge, perineal infection, difficulties in micturition and urinary tract infection. The major problems with these are in the immediate postoperative phase and will be managed under hospital care. Lesser degrees of all these symptoms occur in the weeks subsequent to surgery. Vaginal granulation tissues will give rise to abdominal pain and to tenderness and bleeding on coitus. The pararectal bruising may spread to the ischiorectal fossae. Infection will produce pain, which will not resolve if an abscess forms. Occasionally a missed perineal suture gives rise to localised pain and tenderness. It is therefore important for patients to be advised that healing takes 6 weeks and that the postoperative period is associated with offensive discharge and difficulty in finding a comfortable resting position. Postoperative sexual counselling about scar tenderness, change in the size and direction of the vagina and the understandable defensive lack of libido should be given. Restoration of sexual intercourse will not damage the repair, and the assumption that delay in resumption of coitus will reduce the patient's initial apprehension and discomfort is usually unfounded – rather, she should be gently encouraged to resume intercourse once healing is confirmed 6 to 8 weeks postoperatively.

Unfortunately, some women will have persistent pain following the operation. Surgical incision of the paracervical tissue results in varying degrees of postoperative parametritis, with its associated backache which takes 6 to 8 weeks to resolve. A few women will have scar tenderness due either to excessive fibrotic reaction or to midvaginal stenosis, which may need surgery. Occasionally a small band of adhesion occurs between the anterior and posterior vaginal wall incisions, and this requires division. These difficulties are not related to the degree of prolapse at the initial operation. There is the adage that the worse the prolapse and its associated disturbance of micturition, discomfort and sensation of a lump the less likely it is that minor imperfections following surgery will give rise to significant complaint.

Uterine Malposition

The normal position of antiflexion and anteversion is depicted in Fig. 6.1. The uterus is retroverted in 10 % of women who are basically free of symptoms. It is mobile and capable of anteversion, although it will immediately return to its natural retroverted position. Secondary fixed retroversion is a distinct entity, and the associated pain is due primarily to pathological change, whether inflammatory or endometriotic. In the past all retroversions were considered abnormal, whereas now only a small proportion of uteri with primary retroversion are considered to be the origin of pelvic pain. Differences in the perception of abnormality are attributable in part to an imprecise grading system.

Fig. 6.2 shows a normal-sized uterus with an anteflexed contour lying in the posterior half of the pelvic cavity. A uterus in this position will often rest on the rectum. Anteflexed retroposition is likely to be associated with early vault prolapse and indicates laxity of the uterine support ligaments. It may also be associated with some obstruction of venous return to the broad ligament and the varicose distended vessels that can be seen on laparoscopy or with high-resolution scanning.

The more acutely retroflexed retroverted uterus (Fig. 6.3) will press on the rectum, or by causing the cervix to impinge on the urethra, will initiate urinary hesitancy or, in the extreme, retention of urine. If the ovaries prolapse into the pouch of Douglas significant dyspareunia will ensue. There is also obstruction to venous return with varicosities of vessels in the broad

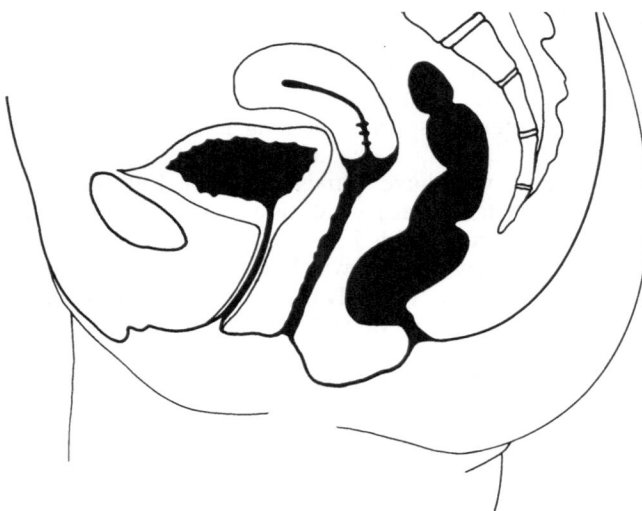

Fig. 6.1. The anteflexed anteverted uterus.

ligament. Both anteflexed retroposition (Fig. 6.2) and retroflexed retroversion (Fig. 6.3) are associated with an increased prevalence of multifollicular change in the ovaries, increasing the tendency to pain. It is important to realise, however, that retroflexion of the uterus and a palpable ovary with ultrasound changes can also be found in symptom free women.

Diagnostic problems can result during the course of routine pelvic examination for contraception and cervical cytology. The examination may reveal a firm swelling in the pouch of Douglas which, if single, has to be differentiated from the fundus of a retroflexed or retroposed uterus. The fundus of a retroflexed or retroposed uterus tends to feel larger than its anteverted counterpart. It is therefore important to obtain an accurate estimate of the size of any swelling in the pelvis, and the knowledge that the transpelvic bony diameter can vary from 10 to 12 cm gives an excellent guideline to such assessment. The pain may be premenstrual in addition to secondary dysmenorrhoea. The pain may be constant or intermittent and associated with dragging in the groin. It is not usually related to exercise, micturition, defaecation or diet and is not relieved by rest. Additionally, low sacral backache may coexist. Varying degrees of rectal pressure, at worse tenesmus, may be present, and a common complaint is difficulty in sitting in one position comfortably, particularly on car journeys.

Uterine malposition can also cause dyspareunia, which can be immediate or postcoital and can persist for 1 to 2 days. A change in menstrual pattern

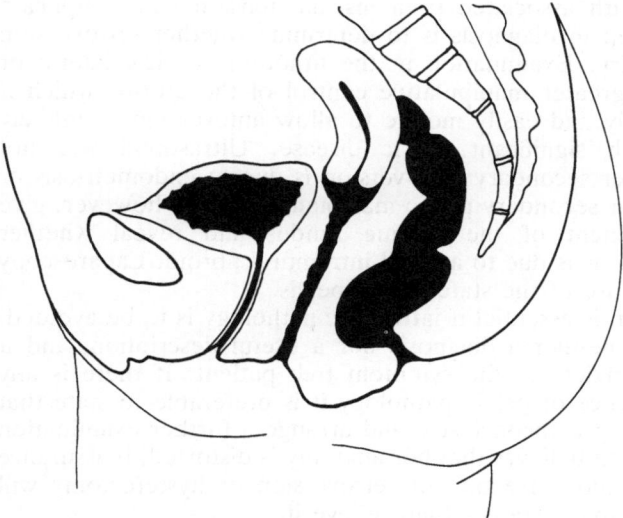

Fig. 6.2. The anteflexed retroposed uterus.

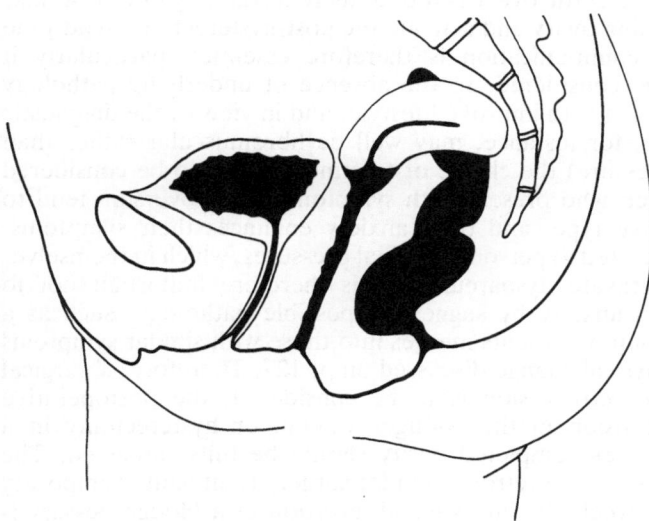

Fig. 6.3. The retroverted retroflexed uterus.

and volume of loss with associated premenstrual tension will complicate diagnosis. The first step in diagnosis is to determine whether retroversion is primary or secondary. Examination in the lithotomy or left lateral or Sims' position allows greater manipulative control of the uterus, which if shown to be sufficiently and easily mobile to allow anteversion is unlikely to be associated with significant pelvic disease. Ultrasound will not readily indicate whether secondary retroversion is due to endometriosis or inflammatory disease or secondary pelvic malignancy. It will, however, give an accurate measurement of the uterine fundus and reveal whether enlargement of the uterus is due to a small intramural fibroid. Laparoscopy will give a clearer picture of the state of the pelvis.

Clear communication is essential if iatrogenic pathology is to be avoided. The "tilted womb" is neither a diagnosis nor a useful description, and it induces unnecessary anxiety in the symptom free patient. If there is any doubt about the existence of pelvic pathology it is preferable to state that the primary examination is inconclusive and arrange a further examination and scan. Once a woman believes that her anatomy is distorted, reassurance will have little effect and correction of retroversion or hysterectomy will merely change the complaint rather than relieve it.

The management of a woman in whom a primary cause is detected will depend on her age and whether she wants more children. Medical management of endometriosis and recurrent pelvic infection is much improved. Excision surgery should be undertaken only after conservative methods have failed. Hysterectomy alone may fail to relieve the symptoms, and bilateral salpingo-oophorectomy will produce an immediate menopause.

Women without significant pelvic disease but with associated menstrual change are usually aged 35 or more, and hysterectomy has many advantages for them. However, if a cystic ovary is found, its removal may induce similar changes in the remaining ovary and activate the post-hysterectomy syndrome (see p. 125). Good communication is therefore essential, particularly if hysterectomy is to be considered. In the absence of underlying pathology the purpose of treatment is to improve lifestyle, and in view of the diagnostic difficulties (backache, for instance, may well be fibromuscular rather than caused by uterine pressure) the choice of treatment needs to be considered very carefully. Women who present with symptomatic retroversion tend to be of the introspective type, and their anxiety enhances their symptoms. The anxiety may be related to personal familial pressures, which in themselves may produce or aggravate dyspareunia. It is therefore important not to increase the patient's anxiety by suggesting possible pathology, such as a cystic ovary. This group of patients merges into those with similar symptoms and no detectable physical change discussed on p. 127. Therefore, if surgical correction of uterine retroversion is to be considered, the postoperative effects of ventrisuspension in the younger woman or hysterectomy in a woman over 35 who has completed parity should be fully discussed. The assessment of primary uterine retroversion for surgery is difficult. Temporary correction for 6 to 8 weeks by intravaginal insertion of a Hodge pessary is unreliable. Spontaneous reversion of the uterus with or without misplacement of the pessary is common but may still be associated with relief of symptoms while the pessary is in the vagina and possible recurrence of symptoms when the pessary is removed. Gynaecological experience is the best guide for surgical intervention in a group of women who will have been subjected to numerous examinations and may be particularly susceptible to agree to surgery.

Pelvic Inflammatory Disease

Pelvic inflammatory disease of the Fallopian tubes, uterus and rarely the ovaries has a wide spectrum of presentation. It may be asymptomatic and discovered incidentally during the course of investigation for infertility, or it may be symptomatic of major pelvic peritonitis. The first attack of primary infection is characterised by general malaise, bilateral lower abdominal pain with secondary nausea and some vomiting and some disturbance of micturition with associated vaginal discharge. There is bilateral lower abdominal tenderness, fever, tenderness in the pouch of Douglas and pain on moving the cervix and uterus. A distinct swelling is rare on the first occasion. Response to antibiotic therapy is good, and only about 15 % of patients will have recurrent attacks. The aggressive coliform septicaemia is fortunately rare and is associated either with menstruation or with pelvic surgery. The classical acute case requires early effective antibiotic treatment (see p. 39).

The diagnosis of pelvic inflammatory disease is summarised in Table 6.1. Laparoscopy offers the possibility not only of accurate bacterial culture but also of excluding other pelvic disease, i.e. appendicitis in the younger woman (on the right side) and diverticulitis in the older woman (on the left). Both are unilateral rather than the bilateral disease associated with salpingitis. With increasing severity secondary pelvic peritonitis occurs, and laparotomy

Table 6.1. Pelvic inflammatory disease: investigations

1. Haemoglobin, white blood cell count, erythrocyte
    sedimentation rate.
    VDRL (blood culture)
2. Bacterological culture (on appropriate medium)
    on samples from:
    Cervix
    Urethra (Mouth)
    Vagina (Rectum)
    + Laparoscopy samples
3. Ultrasound
4. Laparoscopy→laparotomy

may be the only way of ensuring safe management. The need is for analgesia, usually an opiate, adequate fluid intake and a broad spectrum of treatment, namely erythromycin or a tetracycline and metronidazole.

In practice the patient will be admitted to hospital. The real problem of management arises with the suspect and recurrent cases. The suspect cases will have a short history of 3 to 7 days, often postmenstrual, with irregular bleeding and lower abdominal pain. Vaginal discharge and dyspareunia, frequency of micturition, and rectal pressure and backache are all of low degree. Examination reveals a woman who is uncomfortable rather than ill, with a low-grade fever and abdominal and pelvic tenderness without guarding or significant cervical excitation. Laparoscopy will exclude ectopic gestation and endometriosis and will allow swabs to be taken from the Fallopian tubes and pouch of Douglas for bacteriological examination. This is important because sexual transmission of infection is likely, and inadequate or inappropriate antibiotic therapy may mask the infection and lead to recurrence of symptoms and silent Fallopian lumen obstruction.

Laparoscopy is not without risk, and in many cases management is based on the results of the bacteriology of the cervix and the urethra. The ability of broad-spectrum antibiotics to produce a response in 48 hours again makes it difficult to criticise empirical treatment. The less acutely ill patients who are managed at home should be admitted to hospital if the response is not rapid. Women who are not concerned to preserve their fertility can be managed more conservatively. Total healing may take several weeks.

The recurrent cases are either repetitively sexually transmitted or secondarily infected because of an underlying tubal block producing hydrosalpinx (which when infected becomes a pyosalpinx). The intervals between attacks may be from several weeks to months. A common cause for misdiagnosis is bleeding into the pouch of Douglas from an ovarian follicle or retrograde menstruation. The blood alone will cause pain and tenderness for about 12 to 24 hours unless the slight intraperitoneal loss persists. Laparoscopic aspiration of blood-stained fluid from the pouch of Douglas brings rapid relief, but it cannot prevent recurrence. It does, however, offer the possibility of accurate diagnosis.

The recurrent cases can proceed to a true pelvic abscess rather than a contained pyosalpinx. The former requires dependent drainage and the latter excision. Drainage of a pyosalpinx may be effective temporarily, but it is unlikely to leave a normally functioning Fallopian tube capable of ovum transfer.

Chronic pelvic inflammatory disease is associated with lower abdominal pain and groin discomfort which persists and may radiate to the inner aspects of the thigh. Backache and dyspareunia are also noted. There is an association with sterility. Examination will reveal changes from some suspicion of thickening in the lateral fornices to a distinct extrauterine swelling which may vary in size, to be palpable in the pouch of Douglas alone, or a pelviabdominal swelling extending to the umbilicus. The latter is usually due to bilateral hydrosalpingitides. The degree of tenderness will vary with the extent of active inflammatory change. Differential diagnosis due to endometriosis with secondary infection or ovarian malignancy has to be considered.

Table 6.2 lists the common causes of primary and secondary pelvic inflammatory disease. The importance of good communication with a bacteriological colleague has already been emphasised. Whether the patient should be at home or in hospital for the investigations depends on the local circumstances and the severity of the clinical syndrome.

The primary attack of pelvic inflammatory disease will usually respond to antibiotic treatment with erythromycin or terramycin or cotrimoxazole and metronidazole. Consideration of association with a sexually transmitted disease such as gonorrhoea cannot be overemphasised. Failure to respond to treatment or subsequent attacks require hospital admission; laparoscopy should confirm the diagnosis and will allow intrapelvic bacteriological specimens to be taken for culture.

Subsequent discussion should include the prevention of sexually transmitted infection due to coitus, which can occur from adhesion of bacteria to spermatozoa, from the suction effect of coitus introducing organisms into the pouch of Douglas via the uterus and Fallopian tubes and from enhancement of bacterial growth in the vagina by the contraceptive pill. Symptomatic relief under treatment can occur within 2–3 days, but complete healing may take up to 6 weeks. It is therefore worth considering the use of a condom as a barrier to the sexual transmission of reinfection for 3 months. Pelvic inflammatory disease tends to be overdiagnosed, and laparoscopic investigation confirms only about 60 %–70 % of cases considered to be primary pelvic inflammatory disease. Nevertheless the guidance outlined is not unreasonable, particularly if the patient's symptoms are associated with urethritis in the partner.

Recurrence of infection may be due to incomplete healing or reinfection, and sexual habit plays a considerable part in the aetiology. A pragmatic approach is effective if the diagnosis is correct. There is an excellent

Table 6.2. Infective agents in pelvic inflammatory disease

Primary Infection	Organism	Secondary
✓	Gram positive and Gram negative organisms	✓
✓	*Neisseria gonorrhoeae*	
✓	*Mycoplasma, Ureaplasma*	
✓	*Chlamydia trachomatis*	
✓	Anaerobic organisms	✓
✓	*Haemophilus influenzae* (and other oral pathogens)	✓
✓	Herpesvirus	✓
✓	Papilloma wart virus	✓
	Actinomycoses	✓
	Tuberculosis	✓
✓	*Trichomonas vaginalis*	
	Candida	✓

correlation with pelvic inflammatory disease if lower abdominal pain and tenderness and adnexal tenderness, cervical excitation pain and rebound tenderness is elicited. In addition there should be one of the following: mainly fever, leucocytosis, peritoneal purulent material on laparoscopy, vaginal discharge and subsequent positive culture (the latter being present in 20 %–40 % of cases). As mentioned, laparoscopy without bacteriology will give the diagnosis in only 60 %–65 % of cases. Patients with a significant history and confirmatory clinical signs will if treated early be among the 85 % in whom recurrence is unlikely.

Chronicity of pelvic inflammatory disease results in two distinct management problems. The first group are patients with pain and varying degrees of pelvic or pelviabdominal masses which are due to varying stages of fibrotic thickening of the Fallopian tubes and ovaries and their adhesion either to the posterior wall of the uterus, the posterior leaf of the broad ligament or the lateral pelvic wall. Closure of the fimbrial end of the Fallopian tube would be asssociated with distension of the tube by clear fluid or purulent exudate, which eventually is aseptic. In addition, there is the effect of repeated surgical intervention for pelvic peritonitis with or without pelvic tubo ovarian abscess, which makes subsequent conservative surgery unsatisfactory. Discomfort will not be relieved until total pelvic clearance has been performed. It is understandable that there is a reluctance to consider such surgery, but uterine and ovarian conservation is only valid if the option of future in-vitro fertilisation is required. The rare possibility of actinomycotic or tuberculous infection causing chronic pelvic abscess has to be considered and, if appropriate, investigated by culture and histological examination. Both these conditions are amenable to drug treatment, which will also increase the safety of any surgery that may be subsequently indicated. The other group are those patients who are virtually free of symptoms and are discovered during the course of investigation for infertility.

Endometriosis

Endometriosis is a pathological condition due to aberrant siting of endometrial glands, which respond to cyclic hormonal change by bleeding. It is therefore related mainly to the reproductive era, the mean age at diagnosis being 35 years. The duration of presymptomatic endometriosis depends on the extent of the ectopic endometrium and the amount of bleeding. The cause is likely to be a combination of metaplasia of coelomically derived tissue reacting as endometrium, endometrial implantation due to retrograde menstruation, endometrial embolisation via the pelvic lymphatics or pelvic veins and direct implantation following surgery, particularly in pregnancy. Endometriosis appears to have an increasing prevalence in Western centres of up to 2 % of the female population, but the highest rate is among the infertile. Adenomyosis is probably due to direct extension of endometrial tissue into

Table 6.3. Pathology of endometriosis

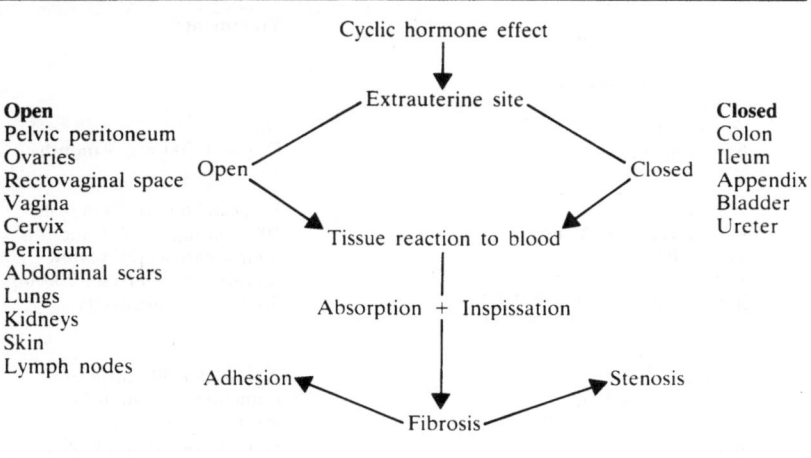

the myometrium, and it may be separate or coexist with pelvic endometriosis.

Table 6.3 indicates the sites of endometriosis. Microscopic bleeding may be resolved within the 4 week cycle. If not, such blood and its reaction will accumulate. The bleeding in an abnormal site, whether open or closed, produces a sterile inflammatory reaction. If the volume of accumulated blood is large enough tissue disturbance will become apparent, and in sites such as the colon or ureter, fibrosis will also produce a stenosis with obstructive symptoms. Tissue adhesion occurs and secondary infection in the pelvis is not unusual.

Table 6.4 classifies endometriosis according to severity and indicates appropriate treatment. The symptoms closely reflect the physical signs, and the severity of pain is related more to the site than to the extent of disease. Untreated, endometriosis spreads progressively and natural remission takes place only with the menopause. Damage due to fibrosis and adhesion resolves slowly, but stenosis is likely to produce partial or complete obstruction. Obstruction of the sigmoid colon in a 50 year-old woman will often be diagnosed as a carcinoma until the histological report is available. Coexistence with fibroids is common. Thyroid autoantibodies and a low or borderline free thyroxine level have also been reported.

Table 6.5 lists the symptoms of endometriosis. Pain starting before or after the onset of menstruation and improving after cessation of menstrual loss with cyclic recurrence is the classic symptom. As the condition extends pain remains throughout the cycle, with exacerbation at menstruation and finally constant severity at all times. Menstrual change is common in endometriotic tissue, and bleeding may be visible when it extends to external

Table 6.4. Classification of endometriosis

Type		Treatment
Mild	Small peritoneal surface lesions	
	Asymptomatic	Nil
	Symptomatic	Danazol 200 mg 3 months
Moderate		
	Ovarian endometrioma < 3 cm	Progestogens or Danazol 600–800 mg for 6–9 months,
	Periovarian ⎫ Peritubal ⎬ adhesion	then laparoscopic review followed by Danazol 200 mg
	Endometrioma: ⎰ peritoneum ⎱ bowel surface	3 months if necessary
Severe		
	Ovarian endometrioma 3 cm +	Age under 30: surgical reduction + 9 months
	Severe adhesion ± tubal obstruction	artificial temporary menopause. Age 31–39:
	Obliteration of pouch of Douglas	depends on severity and clinical need. Age over 40:
	Bowel, urinary tract	pelvic clearance.

sites such as the vagina or perineum. Dyspareunia and bladder and rectal irritability are also common.

Abdominal examination will reveal tenderness if endometriotic leakage has occurred, and a firm tender swelling will be palpable if the ovary is enlarged or the uterus contains an adenomyotic swelling. The results of pelvic examination will vary from no detectable abnormality to a fixed retroversion with tender pelvic nodulation or a large abdominopelvic tumour mass. Retroversion of the uterus is reported in 30 %–55 % of cases. Ultrasound and laparoscopy complete the diagnostic procedures that will differentiate endometriosis from chronic pelvic inflammatory disease, ovarian cysts and uterine fibromyomata. The occasional acute presentation, due to rupture of an endometriotic cyst, gives all the symptoms and signs of an acute lower abdomen.

Table 6.5. Symptoms of endometriosis

Dyspareunia
Painful menses
Constant pain
Menstrual changes
Backache
Infertility
Non-uterine cyclical bleeding

Smaller sites situated on the sigmoid or ileum may mimic regional ileitis or ulcerative colitis. The range of diagnoses varies from asymptomatic endometriosis discovered during the investigation of infertility to endometriotic sites not related to the site of pain. The combination of right iliac fossa pain and left uterosacral endometriosis is not unusual. The more severe forms with nodulation are readily diagnosed on laparoscopy. Lower-bowel or ureteric stenotic endometriosis may be present without ovarian or pelvic forms and may escape diagnosis (despite many years of consultation and investigation) until partial or complete obstruction occurs.

The patient with endometriosis may have difficulty in understanding or accepting the concept of endometrial bleeding from ectopic sites. In addition the prodromal phase may have lasted several years, during which such diagnoses as pelvic infection, cystitis, spastic colon and anxieties may have been suggested. Clinical diagnosis without visual confirmation is unreliable. Once the diagnosis is made enough time must be given to explaining the nature of the disorder to both husband and wife. The purpose of therapy is to arrest endometrial bleeding and allow natural repair. Surgery will be needed for the more extensive lesions, particularly those involving the ovary. Discussion should include the patient's understandable fear of internal bleeding and her concern about her future fertility. The miscarriage rate is higher among untreated women with endometriosis but is reduced by half after treatment. Even after treatment the total pregnancy rate is only 25 %–50 % and is related to the severity of the disease.

The visual appearance ranges from small bluish or black areas of only 1–2 mm diameter to larger swellings which may eventually coalesce to fill the pelvis. These larger areas are usually streaked with chocolate-coloured material, which is inspissated blood. The capsule of the swelling may appear bluish because of its contained inspissated blood.

Medical treatment (with a progestogen or danazol) relies on the inhibition of cyclic bleeding which will allow total resorption of blood and, in most cases, atrophy of endometrial glands. The ensuing artificial menopause should last from 3 to 9 months, the average being 6 to 9 months. It often begins after surgical reduction of the disease in the ovaries. Drug treatment is usually with a progestogen, whose dosage has to be increased stepwise to avoid breakthrough bleeding. Danazol may require 800–1000 mg a day to inhibit loss, though with the minor degrees of endometriosis 200 mg daily can be effective Both progestogens and danazol have unwanted side-effects (Table 6.6). All progestogens are associated with weight gain and may enhance the reactionary depression that already exists. Side-effects of danazol, which are dose dependent, include weight gain, a greasy skin and acne-like eruptions. Treatment is also possible with daily subcutaneous or intranasal inhalation of a luteinising hormone releasing hormone (LHRH) agonist, which can resolve endometric lesions. All these treatments will produce androgenic effects as well as menopausal flushes. They are expensive to maintain and should not be used until the diagnosis is proven. Many patients with endometriosis are desperate enough to attend for daily injections for several months or instil the drugs intranasally at four-hourly

Table 6.6. Effects of drugs used in treatment of endometriosis

Progestogens	*Danazol*
Sensitivity	Contraindicated in pregnancy
Thromboembolism	Foetal androgen effect
Breast cancer	Porphyria
Hepatic insufficiency	Fluid retention
Hypertension	Potentiates anticoagulants
Sodium retention/oedema	Acne
Mastodynia	Hirsutism
Galactorrhoea	Virilisation
Fine hand tremors	Rashes
Sweating	Nervousness
Cramps in calves	Headaches/dizziness
Cholestatic jaundice	Muscle pain
Epilepsy ↑	Hair loss
Migraine ↑	

Arrows indicate increasing severity.

intervals five times a day. Follow-up may require repeat laparoscopy, and treatment has often to be repeated several times.

The more advanced cases with palpable masses will require primary surgery, the extent of which will depend on the patient's age and her desire to have children. Resolution will occur if bilateral oophorectomy is included in the operation, but this will induce a marked menopause which, if treated with cyclic hormones, may cause a recurrence of symptoms. The majority of the gynaecologically extensive cases have mainly ovarian endometriotic cysts with or without obliteration of the pouch of Douglas. Surgery can be difficult and hazardous to bowel and ureter, since the normal anatomical planes are disturbed by the disease and its adhesions. It is therefore necessary to discuss pelvic clearance before any operative procedure. Fortunately, for patients with lesser degrees of ovarian involvement total hysterectomy will resolve the menstrual symptoms, the pain and the dyspareunia.

Up to 7 % of patients will have an ovarian recurrence necessitating further surgery. For younger patients who hope to have children a conservative approach is justified, particularly with the advent of in-vitro fertilisation providing a possibility of pregnancy. Obstruction of the ureter and bowel requires resection and reanastomosis or ureteric implantation. Secondary endometriosis in abdominal scars may be difficult to remove surgically because the margin of the ectopic tissue cannot be defined readily. If necessary, superficial radiation can be used to ablate functioning endometrial glands. Similarly, ovarian ablation with radiotherapy may be safer than a third or fourth laparotomy. Once surgery is indicated, the full implications for the patient should be carefully discussed.

Genital Tract Tumours and Pelvic and Abdominopelvic Swellings

Gynaecological causes of pain are related to the classic pathological subdivisions of congenital anomaly, inflammatory change, neoplasia or trauma. In addition there are anomalies associated with pregnancy and endometriosis. The proximity of all the intrapelvic organs in their peritoneal envelopes and the encircling fibromuscular and bony cage can make identification of the pathological site difficult. Anomalies of pregnancy and endometriosis are often associated with secondary inflammatory change, producing variable swelling that changes according to the response to infection. In the absence of acute episodes related to infection, intraperitoneal bleeding, torsion of tumour pedicles or bleeding into the confines of a tumour, pain may be a late component in presentation. Ovarian cysts and uterine fibromyoma are often discovered as a result of routine examination. Lower abdominal or pelvic discomfort will also depend on individual reaction, and frequently after the chance detection of a swelling the woman will recall that vague pelvic discomfort has been present for months or years.

Table 6.7 lists the common causes of acute onset of symptoms, some of which have already been considered, namely infection (p. 109), pregnancy (p. 69) and endometriosis (p. 112). The most common tumours are those arising in the ovaries and uterus. Large fimbrial or true parovarian cysts do occur, but their presentation does not differ significantly from that of ovarian tumours. Surgical removal of fimbrial or true parovarian cysts is relatively

Table 6.7. Causes of pain in abdominopelvic swellings

Infection	
Primary infection	– Pyosalpinx – Pelvic abscess
Secondary infection	– Post miscarriage/partum
	– Postoperative
	– Appendicitis
	– Intrauterine contraceptive device
Pregnancy	
Ectopic	
Miscarriage	
Fibroid degeneration	
Placental abruption	– Idiopathic
	– Trauma
Endometriosis	
Rupture	
Tumours	
Ovaries	– Pedicle torsion
	– Bleeding
	– Rupture
Uterus	– Tumour degeneration
	– Haematometra, pyometra

simple and rarely involves oophorectomy. Benign ovarian follicles and corpora lutea are rarely more than 5 cm in diameter and will resolve within 4 to 6 weeks. Bimanual pelvic examination in a thin woman is reliable, but persistent swellings or inconclusive examination will require further investigation with ultrasound. Age has an important bearing on the diagnosis, so that an adolescent or woman aged over 35 must be accurately screened in order not to miss malignant ovarian neoplasia. Because of the ovarian pedicle, torsion of cysts up to 10 cm in diameter is more likely, and asymptomatic cysts should be treated as a matter of urgency.

The larger cysts rarely undergo torsion or do so more slowly and less acutely. Pain is therefore not a major factor in the majority of ovarian cysts. The malignancy rate for ovarian cysts is about 10 % in the under-30 age group and rises rapidly with each decade to 60 %–70 % of all ovarian tumours by the 60th year. Unfortunately the majority are seen with secondary spread and poor prognosis. Intracapsular stage 1 ovarian cancer has an 80 % chance of 5-year survival, so early diagnosis is imperative.

Great attention needs to be paid to vague lower abdominal discomfort in women aged over 35, for pelvic tumours rarely cause significant pain. Pelvic swellings of more than 6–8 cm are often associated with vague "indigestion". Bimanual examination should detect the majority of swellings of this size if the lower pole is in the pouch of Douglas. Swellings of less than 8 cm, can be difficult to detect, particularly in the obese. The general outline of the swelling can usually be defined, but its consistency depends on its tension, and differentiation between a tense ovarian cyst and a softened fibroid may not be possible. The abdominal swelling that is separate from the uterus may be a pedunculated fibroid, but such a finding is much more likely with ovarian tumours. Palpation of a well-defined pelvic swelling separate from a normal uterus is a classic finding with ovarian tumours. Only 10 % of benign tumours are bilateral, whereas malignant tumours are rarely unilateral, partly because vague symptoms lead to late diagnosis.

The multinodular abdominopelvic swelling not separate from the uterus feels totally different. Diagnosis then involves the exclusion of bowel disease. Clinical diagnosis is made more difficult by obesity, which generally reduces the effectiveness of scanning. The reduction of intracystic resolution may make it difficult to differentiate between true ovarian cysts and endometriosis or fibromyomata. Diagnosis is based on clinical examination, which should be repeated after bowel evacuation. Chronic retention of urine masquerading as an ovarian cyst is rare.

If examination in an obese patient with vague symptoms is indeterminate, a high-resolution scan should be arranged.

The discovery of an ovarian cyst entails surgical removal by cystectomy with ovarian reconstruction or unilateral oophorectomy (which presumes the diagnosis to be benign). This is relatively simple in a woman aged under 35 with a serous cyst, a dermoid or endometriosis. The diagnosis of ovarian malignancy can be difficult, but in a woman aged over 45 a more radical approach can be used if unsuspected malignancy is discovered at operation. The intermediate age group provides the greatest counselling challenge.

The balance between discussing the possibility of total pelvic clearance preoperatively as opposed to giving the information postoperatively is delicate. If the likely diagnosis is malignant change then preoperative counselling and full discussion should take place. Bilateral oophorectomy without hysterectomy is relevant only in the patient with cardiorespiratory anaesthetic problems or if surgery will involve damage to adjoining viscera without the hope of clearance of malignant disease. Table 6.8 lists the possibilities of investigation of ovarian cysts.

In addition to routine blood screening, patients with suspected ovarian cysts should be given a chest X-ray because of the association of effusion particularly with fibromas and to exclude the possibility of a secondary deposit. Ultrasonography is also very useful. Mesodermal sinus tumours and chorioncarcinomas have tumour markers, and Ca 125 is of some diagnostic value in about 80 % of the epithelial carcinomata. Laparoscopy is contraindicated for tumours over 6 cm in diameter but will allow aspiration of a small follicle cyst and, on occasion, biopsy of other small ovarian tumours.

The emotional impact of being told that oophorectomy – whether unilateral, or particularly, bilateral – is needed must not be underestimated. Hormone replacement therapy may be considered in non-hormonally-active ovarian malignancies, and this too should be fully discussed.

Table 6.9 lists benign and malignant ovarian cysts. Cysts in the follicles and the corpora lutea are functional cysts which are not premalignant. Epithelial cysts may either be benign or malignant. Removal of tumours which have a direct oestrogenic effect, such as granulosa cell tumours, may induce a sudden oestrogen withdrawal effect in postmenopausal women.

Table 6.8. Investigation of ovarian cysts

Type of cyst	X-ray	Ultrasound and CT	Blood	Laparoscopy[a]
Follicle	–	+	–	+
Corpus luteum	–	+	–	+
Serous/Pseudomucinous	Chest	+	Ca125	±
Fibromas	Chest	+	–	+
Dermoid (teratoma)	Pelvic/abdominal	+	–	±
Endodermal sinus	Chest	+	Alpha-fetoprotein	±
Chorioncarcinoma	Chest	+	HCG	±
Granulosa cell	Chest	+	–	±
Dysgerminoma	Chest	+	–	±
Arrhenoblastoma	Chest	+	–	±
Endometriosis		±	–	+

CT, computed tomography;
HCG, human chorionic gonadotrophin
[a] For tumours < 6 cm.

Table 6.9. Ovarian cysts

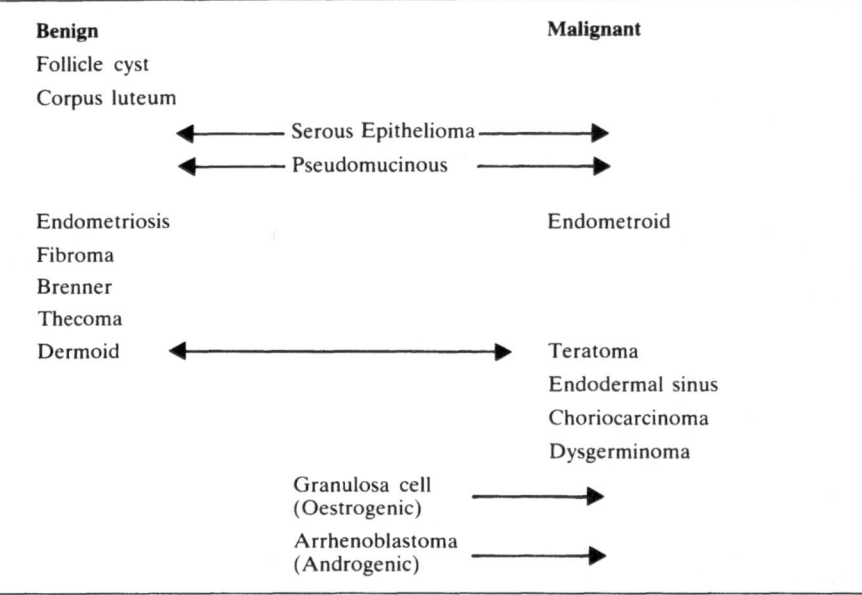

Arrhenoblastomas may have considerable virilising effects. Ovarian endometriosis produces encapsulated cysts containing inspissated blood.

Uterine Enlargement

The uterus enlarges symmetrically in pregnancy unless associated with a bicornuate or double uterus, in which case the side without the gestation sac has a lower growth rate. A similar symmetrical increase in size will result from cervical stenosis producing a haematometra or pyometra and with vaginal obstruction, the haematometra of early adolescence (see p. 62). Asymptomatic enlargement will occur predominantly with fibromyomata (fibroids). Fig. 6.4 illustrates the various sites which, combined with size and rate of growth, produce the noticed clinical changes. Secondary malignant change occurs in about 1 % of fibromyomata. Primary carcinoma of the endometrium rarely produces enlargement beyond 8–10 cm of uterine length, but myometrial sarcoma causes greater enlargement.

The cause of fibromyomata remains unknown. Their association with the reproductive phase and regression following menopause is well documented. The tumour compresses normal myometrium so as to become encapsulated

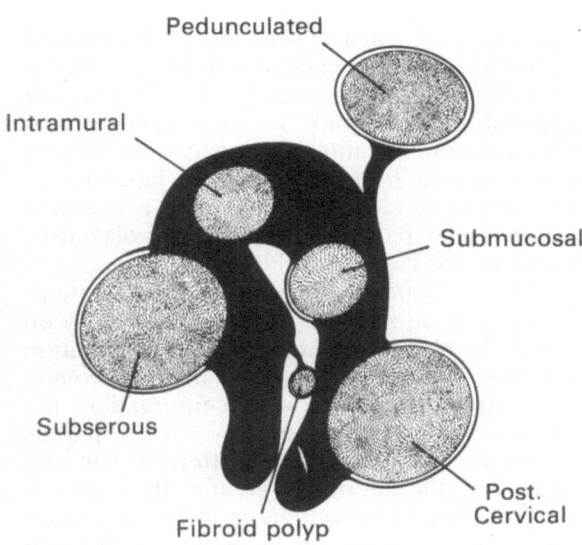

Pedunculated
Intramural
Submucosal
Subserous
Fibroid polyp
Post. Cervical

Fig. 6.4. Sites of "fibroids".

by it, and the histology reveals a fibromuscular structure with varying degrees of degenerative change that have been induced by limitation of blood supply.

A more rapid rate of uterine growth of fibroids can occasionally be induced by oral contraceptives or by progestogens (which are likely to have been used to control menstrual symptoms). An enlarged endometrial cavity will increase menstrual loss, but menorrhagia will also occur in women with either small or large fibroids that have neither distorted nor enlarged the endometrial cavity. The most common cause of excess uterine size is either pregnancy or fibroids, and the two are usually readily distinguishable. Retention of menstrual blood occurs in the young and following cervical surgery and in the elderly due to carcinoma of the endocervix or a senile cervical stenosis producing a pyometra. Menstrual abnormalities both of rhythm and loss are common, as is secondary dysmenorrhoea. Pain of uterine enlargement arises from distention of its peritoneal surface or pressure on adjoining viscera, particularly the bladder and rectum. The pain is progressive with slight variation in intensity, and backache is a feature because the uterus obtains its peritoneal covering from the posterior peritoneal layer. Vascular occlusion or reduction in flow induces necrotic or degenerative change, the intensity of the pain then being directly related to the speed or degree of vascular deprivation.

A uterine fibroid may be impossible to distinguish from an ovarian fibroma not readily separable from the uterus. A pedunculated fibroid can also be misdiagnosed, especially if other uterine fibroids are palpable. The greatest difficulty arises with the combination of fibroids and endometriosis or inflammatory change, a combination more common in West African women than in other groups. Differentiation may be possible only at laparotomy. Enlargements of less than 10 cm should be elucidated by clinical assessment followed by ultrasonography. They rarely require laparotomy for diagnosis. Other causes of uterine enlargement are listed in Table 6.10.

The management of uterine fibroids depends on whether the symptoms are acute or chronic, on age, on parity, on size and site and particularly on secondary effects on viscera such as the bladder or the ureter. The association with parity is indicated by their more frequent diagnosis in infertile women in their later 30s. The choice of treatment is between conservation and observation and surgery by myomectomy or hysterectomy. In the parous woman over 35 years of age, myomectomy has little to offer. If pain and menstrual loss are troublesome and the uterus is greater than 10 cm hysterectomy is the operation of choice. Myomectomy is technically more difficult and freedom from recurrence cannot be assured. Neither can improvement of menstruation. A non-parous woman also aged 35 and recently married with a 15 cm asymptomatic fibroid will be managed by myomectomy. In the non-parous a cervical fibroid may prevent the foetal head from passing through the pelvis, and it can be associated with acute retention of urine by displacing the cervix anteriorly until it occludes the urethra.

Torsion of the pedicle of a fibroid and transcervical extrusion of a fibroid polyp can also cause acute presentation. Torsion of the fibroid pedicle will require laparotomy. A decision as to whether to limit the operation to pedicle division and ligation or to combine it with myomectomy or hysterectomy will have to be made at the time of operation and will be influenced by preoperative discussion and the age and parity of the patient. Extrusion of a pedunculated fibroid polyp of 5–6 cm (and occasionally much larger) through the dilated cervix is usually associated with severe anaemia, often of only 5–6 g/dl. Depending on the degree of extrusion, the fibroid polyp can be removed per vaginam after blood transfusion. Misdiagnosis of

Table 6.10. Causes of uterine enlargement

Pregnancy	
Adenomyosis	
Myohyperplasia	
Fibromyomata	
Carcinoma –	Endometrial
	Cervical
Leiomyosarcoma	
Haematometra	
Pyometra	

a uterine inversion is extremely rare. Gross menstrual blood loss due to fibroids may result in the presentation of severe anaemia and will usually require transfusion before hysterectomy. On occasion an elderly woman is found to have a large abdominopelvic tumour which is firm and may have some irregularity in outline. However, plain X-ray will often show a degree of calcification, and in this instance hysterectomy may not be required if the tumour is asymptomatic. In general, laparotomy is needed to exclude malignancy with certainty.

The guidelines for management must include counselling before hysterectomy, particularly in relation to the discussion of ovarian conservation. Gynaecological surgeons vary in their assessment of the need for hysterectomy. One view is that by always choosing oophorectomy, subsequent silent malignancy is prevented and any problems can be resolved with hormone replacement therapy. The other extreme is not to remove the ovary at any age unless it is associated with recognisable naked-eye pathology. It is important to realise that fibroids of 1–2 cm are common and cause no symptoms and do not always cause pain, menstrual loss or irregularity of cycle. With increasing use of health screening and ultrasonography to detect silent ovarian malignancy, it is important to remember that small fibroids may be associated with symptoms that are in reality caused by some other coexisting disease and should not, without further investigation, be assumed to be the only pathological change requiring treatment.

Pain and discomfort can be relieved with suitable analgesics, and menstrual symptoms as well as pain can be controlled with antiprostaglandins. Various antihacmorrhagics and hormones may relieve the menstrual symptoms, which, however, are likely to recur on cessation of treatment. In certain circumstances a temporary artificial menopause can be induced with progestogens or danazol. Direct medical treatment to reduce the size of fibroids is possible with the luteinising-hormone-releasing-hormone agonist Buserelin by 4-hourly intranasal inhalation. This will produce an artifical menopause and reduce the size of the fibroids but is an expensive treatment best reserved for preoperative reduction of cervical or retroperitoneal fibroids. In summary, once diagnosis has been established for asymptomatic fibroids under 4 cm in diameter all that is required is yearly observation for 3 to 4 years to establish the rate of growth unless anxiety propels the patient towards hysterectomy. The symptomatic relief of pain or menstrual difficulty takes precedence over the size of the fibroids, and hysterectomy is the operation of choice. Myomectomy still has a place for a small group of patients in whom retention of fertility or the prevention of obstructed labour or hazardous Caesarean section is the major consideration.

Post-hysterectomy Pain

Hysterectomy is the commonest major operation in America and Europe. Up to 15 % of women between the ages of 40 and 70 undergo the operation.

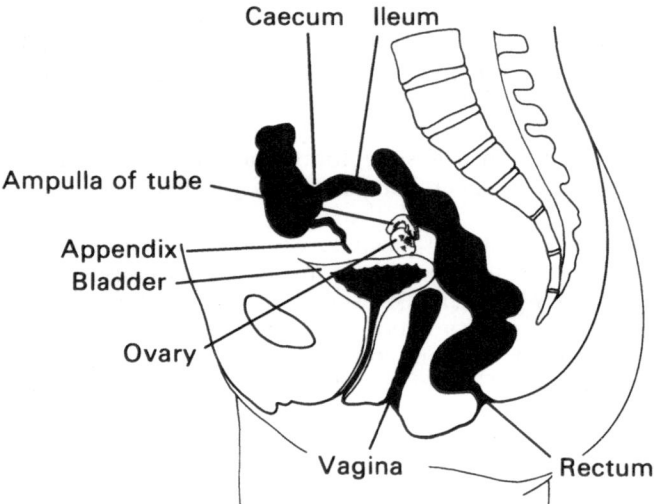

Fig. 6.5. Anatomical relations of the pelvic viscera after hysterectomy.

Fig. 6.5 illustrates the anatomical relations of the pelvic viscera after hysterectomy, particularly the bladder, vaginal vault and rectum. In a population of 100 000 women with a 10 % hysterectomy rate some 300 will develop subsequent follicle cysts, corpora luteal swellings, recurrence of endometriosis, ovarian adhesion and benign and malignant ovarian neoplasia. Some degree of pelvic pain will be present in half of these women, and dyspareunia has been reported in the range of 4 %–65 %. Of those with postoperative pelvic swellings half will require repeat surgery within 5 years. Although a woman can be assured that hysterectomy will give symptomatic relief of menstrual difficulty and menstrual pain, it is important that the risks should be fully considered and discussed preoperatively. The immediate postoperative phase in hospital is associated with varying amounts of pain which are obviously associated with problems such as haematoma formation with infection, particularly parametritis, causing backache and some bowel irritability.

By transecting the upper part of the vagina hysterectomy opens the sterile peritoneal cavity to the normal commensal bacteria of the vagina. The significance of pain is also related to the temperament of the patient. A determined woman may find the postoperative period less uncomfortable than she expected.

The second phase of convalescence, which takes place at home, is accompanied by a varying degree of abdominal wound and lower abdominal discomfort and backache and vaginal discharge. Patients should be advised of the possibility of postoperative urinary tract infection, of difficulties in bowel evacuation and of the fact that relief of pain may occur for 2 or 3 days and then recur. It is helpful to advise that these symptoms and the associated tiredness will resolve gradually but the degree of physical activity tolerated will increase, so that wound discomfort may be induced by half an hour of activity in the second postoperative week but will be noted only after several hours of activity in the 4th and 5th postoperative weeks.

Table 6.11 lists the possible causes of pain which either persists after the 6-week convalescence period or recurs in the ensuing months. Chronic abscess formation will require surgical incision with dependent drainage. Wound herniation is fortunately rare but requires repair, and defects of the rectus sheath, if considerable, may be very difficult to restore. Nerve entrapment in relation to the scar or small areas of anaesthesia can give rise to concern and is unlikely to be resolved by surgical incision unless a distinct spot can be outlined, and even then it could be a referred effect. The services of a pain clinic can be very useful. Endometriosis of the abdominal scar is best dealt with by surgical excision. On occasion it may involve reopening of the peritoneal cavity because of the extension of endometriosis.

The residual ovary syndrome produces considerable problems of management. In essence if there is a palpable or recognisable swelling which persists, then further laparotomy will be necessary. It will require oophorectomy and

Table 6.11. Post-hysterectomy management

Abdominal wall	
Chronic abscess[a]	Incision
Hernia	Repair
Nerve entrapment	Electric stimulation
Endometriosis	Drugs/surgery/radiotherapy
Pelvic cavity	
Residual ovary	Scanning/laparoscopy/surgery
Chronic pelvic abscess or pseudocyst	Surgical
Vesicorectal adhesion	Counselling
Ureteric obstruction	Surgery
Vaginal vault	
Granulation tissue[a]	Cautery
Sexual problems	Counselling
Renal	
Urinary infection	Antibiotics
Incontinence	Investigate
Gastrointestinal	
Constipation	Diet/counselling
Obstruction	Surgery

[a] Unless secondary to underlying pathology.

in the circumstance of ovarian endometriotic change may best be managed by bilateral oophorectomy.

The risk of residual ovarian malignancy is about 1 in 500. The probability of a palpable ovarian tumour being due to malignancy rises with age and the interval since hysterectomy.

Vesicorectal adhesion is of little significance and should not be considered as pathological change requiring surgical intervention. It does, however, produce some changes in sexual experience, and the patient may fear that coitus will cause vault damage. She should be warned that the first phase of resumption of sexual life may be associated with some vault discomfort because of the healing scar that there will be some slight blood loss if granulation tissue is present and that pressure on the bladder (being attached to the vault of the vagina) may induce a feeling of the need to micturate. These experiences will resolve over a period of 2 weeks to 2 months, and the patient should be encouraged to maintain sexual activity in order to desensitise the vaginal vault. Assurance should also be given that the absence of any of these symptoms should not indicate a failure of proper healing. The family practitioner may have knowledge of any prehysterectomy sexual difficulty and should so have advised the gynaecologist. Unrecorded psychosexual problems will persist after hysterectomy.

An additional sexual problem may be that of shortening of the vagina, particularly after radical hysterectomy and its associated dryness as the result of ovarian failure or following bilateral oophorectomy. A woman with normal libido who experiences the effects of a short vagina should be encouraged to maintain a sexual life, since the vagina will lengthen over the course of a year. Vaginal dryness can be relieved with the use of hormone replacement. Oestrogen cream does not have the drawback of induced bleeding or effects on the uterus. Dryness without other menopausal changes may well be due to anxiety and can be relieved with a lubricant rather than with hormone treatment.

Long-term ureteric displacement inducing hydronephrosis is a rare complication of hysterectomy. The persistence of unilateral pain will require investigation with intravenous pyelography which may not show a kinking of the ureter if it has not produced any significant obstruction. The major ureteric problems are usually in the immediate postoperative phase. Improved surgical technique and preoperative preparation have reduced the need for postoperative catheterisation. This has lowered the incidence of postoperative urinary infection which, once it has occurred, has a tendency to recur, requiring bacteriological assessment and suitable antibiotic treatment. Nevertheless some degree of frequency of micturition and nocturia is a problem until the parametrial swelling which occurs after hysterectomy has completely resolved (usually within 3 months). On occasion, a borderline urge incontinence or stress incontinence will be aggravated by hysterectomy. The necessary urodynamic differentiation is advisable so that treatment can be definitive.

Chronic pelvic abscess is very slow to resolve and it may be 6 months to a year before there is complete relief of pain. If there has been any blood in the pouch of Douglas a pseudocyst may form, producing all the clinical characteristics of a cystic swelling which is palpable both vaginally and abdominally. Fortunately a pseudocyst will respond to aspiration, though laparotomy will usually be necessary.

Chronic vaginal vault granulation tissue is a problem in up to 10 % of women following hysterectomy. It is almost always a local reaction of the vaginal mucosa and if of minor degree will respond readily to the application of silver nitrate. However, more profuse granulation tissue or recurrence is best dealt with by diathermy cauterisation under anaesthesia. This also enables an examination under anaesthesia to be performed to exclude a remnant of a chronic abscess or the rare prolapse of the ampullary portion of the Fallopian tube. The latter is more likely to occur 6 to 8 weeks postoperatively than later.

Chronic constipation is a common complaint after hysterectomy. It is important to be sure what is meant. Delay in bowel evacuation and incomplete evacuation are common in the immediate postoperative phase, particularly in women who had prior difficulty with defaecation. If there has been no prior problem and the constipation has not resolved with diet, adequate fluid intake and the short term use of bulk forming drugs and faecal softeners, then investigation for possible bowel disease should be undertaken.

Post-hysterectomy problems may be prevented if total or partial endometrial resection is proven effective management of menstrual excess and so reduces the incidence of hysterectomy.

Gynaecalgia

Although a pathological cause can be identified for most cases of chronic pelvic pain, there remains a small percentage for which no physical cause can be found. To this group of cases without significant pathology is applied the term "gynaecalgia". Factors that may contribute to gynaecalgia are shown in Fig. 6.6. The characteristics of gynaecalgia and the features commonly associated with the disorder are shown in Fig. 6.7. Women with the gynaecalgia syndrome are usually 25 to 40 years of age and have had at least one child. Their symptoms are of at least 2 (and often many more) years' duration, infrequently with an acute exacerbation. The history is indistinct and the siting of pain vague, though usually confined to the lower abdomen, radiating to the groins and to the upper and inner thighs. The language of description is often exaggerated, with terms such as "terrible" or "intolerable", but without a significant change in lifestyle. A wish for a change in lifestyle may, however, be pertinent. Dyspareunia, menstrual change, backache, urinary and bowel disturbance, fatigue and obvious anxiety with depressive elements are common. It is virtually impossible to

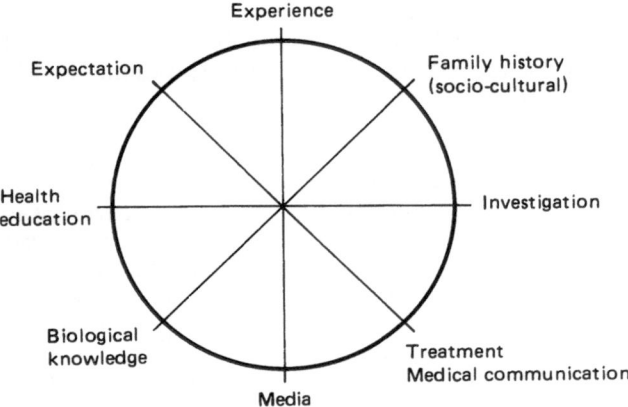

Fig. 6.6. Factors influencing experience of gynaecalgia.

dissociate the anxieties from the other symptoms and often difficult to assess personality and reaction to previous stress of any causation or association. The duration of symptoms is a guide to possible cause, a short history (1 to 4 weeks) pointing to infection – a diagnosis that is confirmed by a good response to early treatment. "Cancerophobia" is a significant cause of anxiety, but malignant change is progressive and the long history eliminates

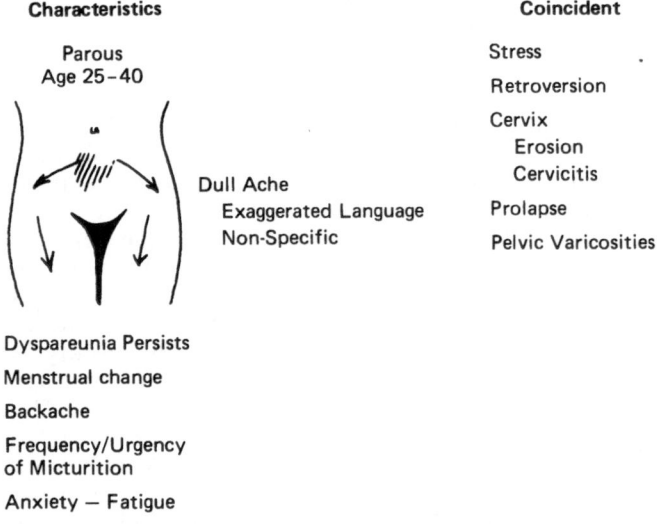

Fig. 6.7. Characteristics of, and features associated with, gynaecalgia.

such a diagnosis unless obscured by recurrent complaint. Persistence of pain without clinical or physical signs may be due to the range of personal and sexual activity and to awareness of reproductive physiology such as ovulation bleeding and premenstrual tension. It is also necessary to consider whether the discovery of uterine retroversion with or without prolapse, chronic cervicitis or cervical erosion is in fact the true cause of pain and not a coincidental finding.

A short history and a quick examination is unproductive, and the extent and timing of investigation will be determined after the initial consultation, particularly if any empirical treatment has failed. In the first 3 to 6 months of complaint, investigation should be non-invasive unless the pain is severe and acute. The sequence of diagnostic investigations should be: clinical examination, bacteriology and cytology, continuing to ultrasonography and rarely computed tomographic scanning. Further investigation includes examination under anaesthesia and surgical laparoscopy. Bladder and bowel problems are more site specific, and investigation will often include a urine culture, pyelography, sigmoidoscopy, colonoscopy and contrast enema radiology. Lumbar sacral and pelvic girdle radiology are also required to exclude bone disease. Generally, these examinations are performed over a period of months or years as one negative result follows another. Nevertheless persistent pelvic pain does result in the full range of investigation, and only in this way can recognisable pelvic disease be excluded.

In 50 % of cases the first consultation for pelvic pain will be sufficiently specific or associated with physical signs. Investigation will support the diagnosis, and specific treatment can be provided. In the residual 50 % the cause may well remain unresolved for many years. Women by their late 40s may have accepted that recurrent investigation has not been helpful, and their pain may have lessened or reduced in significance. There is an increase of such pain in the over-60s, particularly in women living on their own. In such women (after gynaecological disease and bowel malignancy have been excluded) the possibility that diverticulosis is in fact the cause of pelvic pain needs to be considered. It is therefore important not to suggest pathology by name unless there is clear evidence that it is correct. The clinical diagnosis of pelvic inflammatory disease is not substantiated in some 30 %–35 % of women, and neither is the diagnosis of mild endometriosis. Either of these positive diagnoses will need later contradiction if not proven, and this can cause difficulties in management. To explain that investigation is required for diagnosis and deliberately to advise that a diagnosis is not confirmed will prove valueless. The woman who has been told that her "ovaries or tubes" are causing pain finds no relief when they are normal on laparoscopy. The first consultation influences the timing of investigation. The associated discussion can cause management problems if not handled carefully. Armchair advice is easier than the practical management of a distressed couple who have been given several different explanations for the woman's pain without relief and who may already be feeling resentment at the manner in which they have been treated. Repeated attendances at busy hospital clinics tend to accentuate the problem.

Stress due to family or occupation or sexual difficulty in any combination can be difficult to elicit but needs consideration. As always familial and sexual problems may be secondary. Unresolved major or recurrent stress factors may be involved.

Sexual fantasy is rarely volunteered but sexual expectation should be given an opportunity of expression. Fears are described more readily, particularly those related to pregnancy, sexually transmitted disease, unfaithful partners and family history of cancer.

Dieting, and particularly obesity, may indicate a dissatisfaction with femininity, and women with such difficulties need sympathetic counselling and psychological support. The unfortunate women who can maintain a reasonable weight only by stringent dieting are particularly difficult to manage. Withholding advice fairly early in the management of pelvic pain is detrimental to future success. Most women will cooperate if told sympathetically that psychological stress can aggravate pain and that one is trying to give the best practical help. Those who adamantly refuse to participate in psychological support may in fact be enhancing their need for such advice.

The group with disturbances of menstrual loss and/or cycle can be helped by using the combined contraceptive pill with low oestrogen and high progesterone content. The thin non-smoker can safely use such treatment beyond 35 years of age and probably beyond 40.

A temporary menopause with progestogens or danazol for 3 months can also be useful. If the pain is relieved then the problem may have been induced by menstruation and its associated increased blood flow in the broad ligament. Hysterectomy in the over 35s can be considered, but careful counselling should ensure that whereas hysterectomy will prevent any menstrual or contraceptive problem, it cannot be guaranteed to relieve gynaecological pelvic pain, and that in itself hysterectomy has painful sequelae.

Discovery of a retroverted uterus does not indicate that it is the cause of pain, but once the patient is counselled that "the womb is tilted", a request for treatment becomes increasingly difficult to resist. Surgical correction brings its own problems of abdominal pain and frequent relapse to retroversion. A mobile "tender" retroverted uterus of normal size with a laparoscopically clear pelvis does not require surgery.

A similar problem arises with primary cervical erosion with or without secondary cervicitis. The granular red cervix looks unnatural but is common in nulliparae and in pill users. The parous cervix with Nabothian follicles, larger than its nulliparous counterpart, may also be considered abnormal.

The tissue connections of the cervix to the parametrium laterally and the bladder anteriorly can cause bladder irritability, giving frequency, backache and groin pain. There is a stage when cervical cautery will have to be considered. At present it is preferable not to suggest that a nulliparous cervical erosion or parous cervicitis are the cause of pain. Often cauterisation provides temporary healing for 6 months to a year, and a smaller group achieve symptomatic relief. Once advised that a lesion is present, particularly if the word ulcer is used, then cauterisation should be performed with cytology and colposcopy as required.

Pelvic congestion has been considered as a cause of pelvic pain for many years. Varicosities and enlarged veins of the broad ligament have been noted at laparotomy. Modern ultrasonography has shown that these engorged vessels are present in the gynaecalgia syndrome, and confirmation can be obtained by laparoscopy. These investigations also show some enlargement of the ovary with cystic follicular changes, all of which are more common in relation to oestrogen levels. Anti-oestrogens such as danazol and progestogens can be used temporarily or intermittently in the younger women who may wish to conceive subsequently. If relief of pain and reduction of blood flow occurs, then pelvic congestion can be considered to be the aetiological agent.

In hospital practice it is important to establish the complaint for which relief is required. Discussion about the relationship between pain and anxiety is complex, but personal experience is that pain causes anxiety and anxiety accentuates pain. There is a good response to outlining the purpose of investigation and the role of ultrasonography and laparoscopy. Of the 50 % who are with pain and immediately discovered pelvic pathology, half (25 % of the total) will subsequently be found to have changes in the borderline between physiological and pathological significance. In this group, carefully counselled treatment will relieve or improve symptomalogy or at least give comfort. Again time is well spent in explaining that minor problems such as a few spots of endometriosis or an intermittent retroversion are best managed conservatively and are not of serious disease significance. The remainder should have access to pain clinics with the regimens of assistance as outlined in Chapter 8. General physical fitness, ability to sleep, fulfilment of a reasonable percentage of life expectations and the prevention of resentment are important guidelines. Expert psychological support should be given to volunteers for such treatment.

No criticism of attendance at holistic centres, osteopaths or acupuncturists should be implied. For a small number of patients a change in medical adviser is also helpful. As with all human relationships, a difficult patient/ doctor relationship may be improved by a change of practitioner.

7 Surgical and Orthopaedic Causes of Pelvic Pain

D.G. JONES and D.E. STURDY

Surgical Causes of Pelvic Pain

D.E. Sturdy

Acute Intestinal Inflammation

Acute appendicitis, sigmoid diverticulitis, ileal Crohn's disease (regional ileitis) and salpingitis are acute inflammatory disorders within the pelvis which produce both visceral and somatic pain due to involvement of the parietal peritoneum. All these disorders in the acute phase have the following symptoms and physical signs in common:

Lower abdominal pelvic pain (right sided in appendicitis, left sided in diverticulitis)

Nausea and vomiting

Pyrexial flushed patient with furred tongue and halitosis

Tachycardia

Lower abdominal pain intensified by increased abdominal pressure, e.g. by coughing or walking

Tenderness in the inflamed area on rectal or vaginal examination

Hyperactive bowel sounds in the first 48 hours

Absence of bowel sounds when generalised peritonitis develops in 48 hours

In delayed diagnosis localisation of the inflammation produces a tender mass (in the right side in appendicitis, in the left side in diverticulitis). The greater omentum (abdominal policeman) is nearly always involved in localised masses.

Perforation into the peritoneal cavity produces generalised peritonitis

Perforation into the pelvic cavity may produce a residual pelvic abscess

Acute salpingitis can mimic either acute appendicitis or acute diverticulitis, depending on which Fallopian tube is involved. Acute Crohn's disease (regional ileitis) of the ileum and inflammation of a Meckel's diverticulum (Meckel's diverticulitis) closely resemble acute appendicitis in their presentation. Acute lower urinary tract infection may be mistaken for an inflammatory bowel lesion in the female pelvis.

Diagnosis may be difficult in young children and elderly women. Children usually present with vomiting and the abdominal signs appear late. Below the age of 6 years 50 % of acute appendicitis patients will have perforated. Elderly patients appear to have a reduced constitutional response to the inflammatory reaction with the abdominal and pelvic peritoneal cavity, and in 70 % of patients over 60 years of age with appendicitis perforation will have occurred at presentation. Apart from the elderly group nearly all patients will have a polymorphonuclear leucocytosis. A plain abdominal film may show dilated loops of small bowel in proximity to the site of pelvic inflammation. A laparoscopy should not be undertaken in the presence of acute inflammation. When a patient presents with an "acute abdomen" the surgeon should advise an emergency laparotomy despite the absence of a concrete diagnosis. Fig. 7.1 depicts the age incidence of acute pelvic inflammatory disorders in female patients.

The general principles in the treatment of acute inflammatory conditions in the pelvic cavity are emergency removel of the inflamed viscus with drainage of the inflamed area and of the pelvic cavity if indicated.

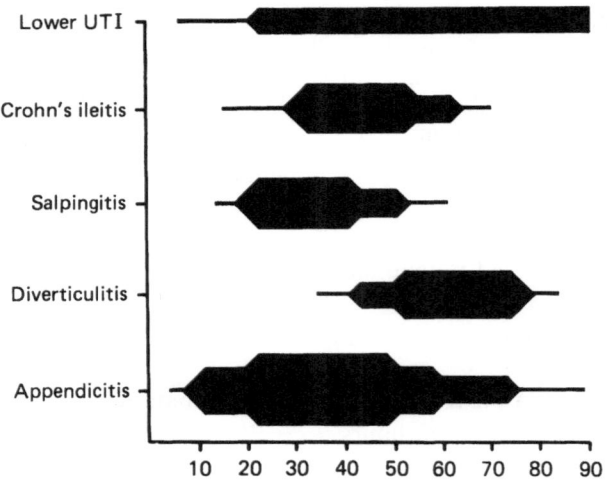

Fig. 7.1. Age incidence of acute inflammation of the female pelvic organs (UTI = urinary tract infection).

Pelvic Abscess

A pelvic abscess is a localised collection of pus in the rectouterine pouch of Douglas (Fig. 1.2) walled off by loops of small intestine and by the greater omentum. A pelvic abscess is a well-recognised complication of acute appendicitis, diverticulitis and salpingitis but may be produced by any intraperitoneal inflammatory condition, by perforation of the bowel or other intra-abdominal viscus or by leakage from a surgical anastomosis. A small proportion of pelvic abscesses are idiopathic in origin.

Persistent postoperative fever, lower abdominal discomfort, mucoid diarrhoea and sometimes frequency of micturition should indicate the possibility of a collection of pus in the pelvic cavity. Rectal examination reveals a tender, boggy swelling anteriorly, and larger abscesses are palpable in the hypogastric region. The patient will have a polymorphonuclear leucocytosis. An ultasound scan of the pelvis may be helpful in diagnosis (Fig. 7.2).

Spontaneous discharge into the rectum or vagina usually occurs in 7 to 10 days. Some abscesses need drainage via the rectum or extraperitoneal suprapubic drainage.

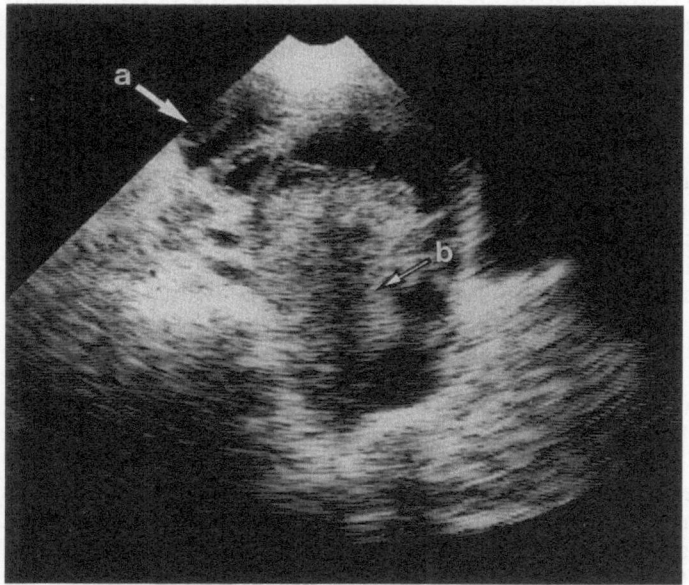

Fig. 7.2. Ultrasound scan of pelvic abscess: **a**, loops of bowel; **b**, abscess.

Acute Intestinal Ischaemia and Obstruction

Both the large and small bowel may become acutely obstructed in the pelvis and lead to the classical symptoms and signs of intestinal obstruction – vomiting, colicky abdominal pain, constipation, abdominal distension and obstructive bowel sounds. Intestinal ischaemia will produce the same symptoms with the exception that the ischaemic bowel is exquisitely tender with rebound tenderness on abdominal examination and tenderness high in the pelvis on vaginal examination. The commonest causes of bowel obstruction in the female are incarceration of a hernia, colonic neoplasm, volvulus, and benign strictures as seen in diverticular disease, Crohn's disease or ulcerative colitis.

Loops of terminal ileum are notoriously prone to become adherent to structures within the pelvis after infection or by adhesion or incarceration within a hernial protrusion, resulting in intestinal obstruction. A more sinister development in the obstructed bowel is ischaemia and necrosis, due either to pressure within a narrow hernial orifice or to a closed-loop volvulus of the bowel. In the latter condition both ends of a loop of ileum are entrapped, and increasing tension within the loop compresses the venous drainage and eventually the arterial supply to the bowel. Strangulation occurs, and the necrotic bowel perforates, producing fulminating and often fatal peritonitis or a pelvic abscess. Treatment of acute obstruction is immediate surgery and relief of the obstruction before the bowel becomes ischaemic and perforates. The ischaemic bowel is resected.

Herniae

Femoral herniae account for 20 % of female hernias. They usually contain terminal ileum and omentum (rarely the bladder) and, because of rigidity of the neck are much more prone to strangulate than the inguinal variety. When a patient presents with chronic pelvic pain the hernial orifices must always be examined for the presence of an inguinal or femoral hernia. Increased pain and increased tension and tenderness within the hernial swelling indicate that incarceration has occurred and that strangulation is imminent. Urgent surgical treatment to release the hernial contents and to repair the hernia is indicated in these patients.

Obturator herniae, which are very rare (though commoner in women than men), protrude through the obturator fossa alongside the obturator vessels and nearly always contain small intestine. Diagnosis is rarely possible until the hernia incarcerates or strangulates, when lateral-wall pelvic pain becomes prominent and in many cases is referred down the medial side of the thigh to the knee along the geniculate branch of the obturator nerve (L2, 3, 4). Immediate operation is indicated for relief of obstruction and closure of the obturator canal defect.

Chronic Inflammatory Bowel Disease

Chronic Appendicitis

The existence of chronic appendicitis as a cause of chronic right sided abdominal pain is debatable. Until the mid 1970s removal of the appendix for chronic lower abdominal or pelvic pain was commonplace, but the results in terms of symptomatic improvement were frequently disappointing. In modern clinical practice a diagnosis of chronic appendicitis is hardly ever justified, except in those patients who have previously had a clinical attack of acute inflammation. In these circumstances appendicectomy cures the patient's chronic pain.

Diverticular Disease

Diverticular disease of the colon (diverticulosis) is an acquired condition which appears in the 5th to 7th decade with equal frequency in the two sexes. A third of the population of the Western hemisphere over 50 years of age will have evidence of asymptomatic diverticulosis of the colon. In 65 % of patients the sigmoid colon alone is involved and, where the rest of the colon exhibits diverticula, the sigmoid colon is also affected by diverticulosis. The rectum is never involved in large-bowel diverticulosis.

Diverticula are produced by increase in intraluminal pressure which causes a protrusion of bowel mucosa alongside the segmental blood vessels and through the circular muscle (pulsion diverticulum) between the mesenteric and antimesenteric taeniae. Constipation with aggregation of scybalous masses in the sigmoid colon is an aetiological factor. In 85 % of patients diverticulosis is asymptomatic. Inflammation of one or more diverticula will produce diverticulitis of varying severity. The complications of diverticulitis are: abscess formation, perforation, haemorrhage, stricture formation and colovesical or colovaginal fistulae. Seventy-five per cent of colovaginal or colovesical fistulae are due to diverticular disease. The remaining 25 % result from a colonic neoplasm. In symptom-free patients diverticulosis is an incidental finding in barium studies of the large bowel for unrelated reasons. Symptoms, when present, are intermittent moderate to severe pain in the left lower abdomen and left side of the pelvis and a feeling of bowel distension. Bowel habit changes, with small hard stools (sheep droppings) or, in some cases, alternating diarrhoea and constipation. Mucus is passed with the stools. Rectal bleeding is rare except in the over-70s, in whom a heavy dark red melaena stool is the presenting symptom. On abdominal examination there is tenderness in the left iliac fossa, and occasionally a mass is palpable in that region. Tenderness high in the left side of the pelvis may be elicited by rectal and vaginal examination with pressure on the cervix. Endoscopy is often unrewarding because of bowel spasm, but diverticula are occasionally seen as red-edged depressions in the sigmoid colon. An air contrast barium enema is diagnostic (Fig. 7.3) and will demonstrate the diverticula with associated spasm of the sigmoid loop. Great care is taken by the radiologist to exclude a coexisting carcinoma of the pelvic colon.

Uncomplicated diverticulosis (80 % of cases) can be managed with a high-fibre diet (including bran), mild laxatives and antispasmodic drugs. Repeated attacks of diverticulitis (15 %) indicate the need for surgical treatment with sigmoid colectomy. Complicated diverticulitis (5 %) will require excision of the diseased bowel, strictures or fistulae.

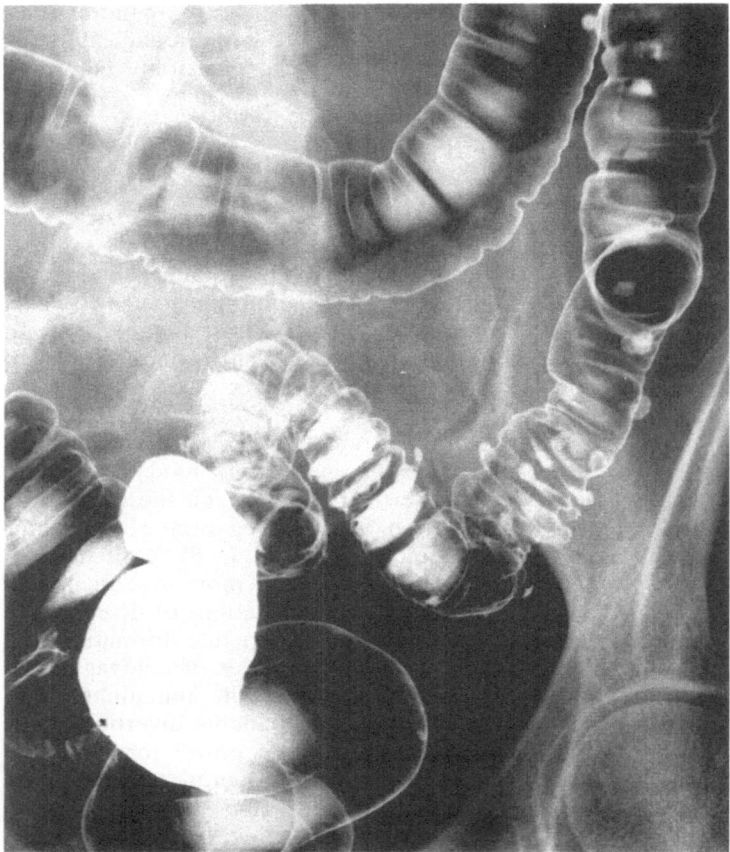

Fig. 7.3. Double contrast barium enema showing diverticulosis.

Crohn's Disease

In the pelvis Crohn's disease may affect the terminal ileum and caecum or the rectum and sigmoid colon. The aetiology of the disorder is unknown. An autoimmune aetiology has been suggested. Crohn's disease is a chronic granulomatous inflammation of *all* layers of the bowel wall and can occur anywhere from the oesophagus to the anus. In the small bowel it characteristically occurs in isolated bowel segments (skip lesions), and intramural fibrosis in these lesions frequently leads to stricture formation. In 60 % of patients the disease is limited to the ileocaecal region. In 20 % the proximal and distal bowel is involved. In 20 % the disease is confined to the colon and rectum.

The complications of Crohn's disease are: stricture formation, intestinal obstruction, perforation, fistula formation and haemorrhage. In 25 % of patients with ileocaecal Crohn's disease perianal abscesses, fissures or fistulae may occur, and in 50 % of patients with colorectal Crohn's disease perianal complications are present. The systemic manifestations of Crohn's disease are: intermittent fever, malaise, anaemia, clubbing of the fingers, arthritis or arthralgia, iritis, erythema nodosum and pyoderma gangrenosum. Compared with the general population, Crohn's disease patients run a slightly higher risk of developing bowel carcinoma.

Ileocaecal Crohn's disease presents as an acute appendicitis or a mass in the right iliac fossa (Fig. 2.4). Large-bowel Crohn's disease is diagnosed by evaluation of the clinical signs and symptoms combined with endoscopic examination of the terminal large bowel and histology of the rectal mucosa or of chronic anal fissures and fistulae. The specific symptoms of large-bowel inflammation are common to those found in ulcerative proctocolitis. Diarrhoea occurs in 80 % of patients, with mucus and occasionally dark red blood. Rectal discomfort and tenderness are common symptoms. Rectal examination usually reveals no abnormality. Sigmoidoscopy will reveal an oedematous inflamed red mucosa covered with a mucoid discharge and occasional patches of haemorrhage. Fissures, fistulae and inflamed skin tags or piles are corroborative evidence of Crohn's disease. In 70 % a biopsy reveals lymphoid aggregates and granulomas. Air contrast barium enema studies may help in diagnosis. The radiological appearances of a rigid bowel with irregular fine fissures (rose-thorn ulcers) are better seen in the transverse and descending colons (Fig. 7.4). In many patients the rectum itself is radiologically normal. Differentiation between Crohn's disease and ulcerative proctocolitis is often difficult on a barium enema examination.

Medical therapy with steroids may effect a temporary improvement. Limited surgical excision or a stricturoplasty is indicated for small-bowel strictures. Obstructing ileocaecal Crohn's disease is treated with a limited right hemicolectomy. Perianal manifestations of Crohn's disease are treated with local excision and packing. Severe rectal involvement demands excision of the rectum and a colostomy. Fifty per cent of patients have a recurrence of Crohn's disease within 5 years of bowel resection, and for this reason primary surgical exicision of bowel must be as limited as is possible.

Ulcerative Proctocolitis

The aetiology of proctocolitis is unknown. Rectal involvement occurs in 95 % of cases, with proximal spread to the colon for a variable distance. The terminal ileum is involved in reflux ileitis in 18 % of cases. In 10 % of patients the rectum and entire colon are involved. Inflammation primarily involves the bowel mucosa, and muscle involvement follows at a later stage of the disease. Five per cent of patients present with an acute fulminating colitis, which may produce a grossly distended large bowel (toxic megacolon) and lead to perforation of the bowel, which in many cases is fatal. Ninety per cent of patients present with chronic proctocolitis. Local complications are: bleeding, perforation, stricture formation, perianal suppuration and (in 15 %) development of a carcinoma after 15 years. Systemic complications

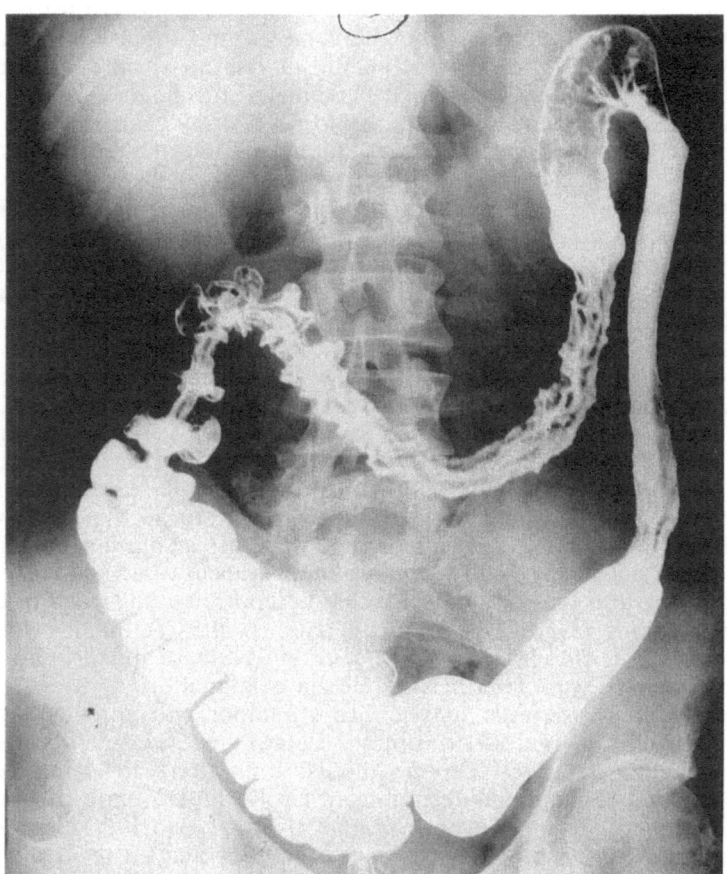

Fig. 7.4. Barium enema study demonstrating Crohn's disease of the transverse colon.

include: arthropathy (25 %) iritis (5 %), dermatoses and liver fibrosis.

In 15 % of patients with chronic ulcerative proctocolitis carcinoma develops approximately 15 years after onset of the disease. Eighty per cent of these carcinomas arise in the rectosigmoid segment of the large bowel and are accessible to digital and endoscopic examination of the rectum.

A diagnosis of ulcerative colitis is made from evaluation of the patient's symptoms combined with endoscopy, biopsy and air contrast barium studies. Inflammation of the rectal mucosa gives rise to tenesmus, rectal pain and pink, bloody, mucoid diarrhoea. Rectal examination reveals a spongy mucosa with pinkish red blood on the examining finger. In 95 % of patients sigmoidoscopy will reveal a red granular mucosa, which bleeds easily even on gentle pressure from a gauze pledget (contact bleeding). Histological examination of a rectal biopsy specimen shows inflammatory changes in the mucosa, but differentiation from Crohn's disease is difficult. An air contrast examination will reveal narrowing and rigidity of the bowel with absence of haustrations and multiple mucosal pseudopolyps (Fig. 7.5)

Chronic inflammatory bowel disease may be due to ulcerative colitis or Crohn's disease, and differentiation is difficult on clinical, endoscopic, radiological and histological grounds. Diagnosis may be aided by reference to Table 7.1.

Acute proctocolitis should be managed initially with systemic steroids, which will control symptoms in 97 % of patients. Relapsing ulcerative colitis, which occurs in 75 % of patients, is treated with oral sulphasalazine and prednisone retention enemas. Fifteen per cent of patients will require surgery, which involves removal of the whole of the large bowel with either

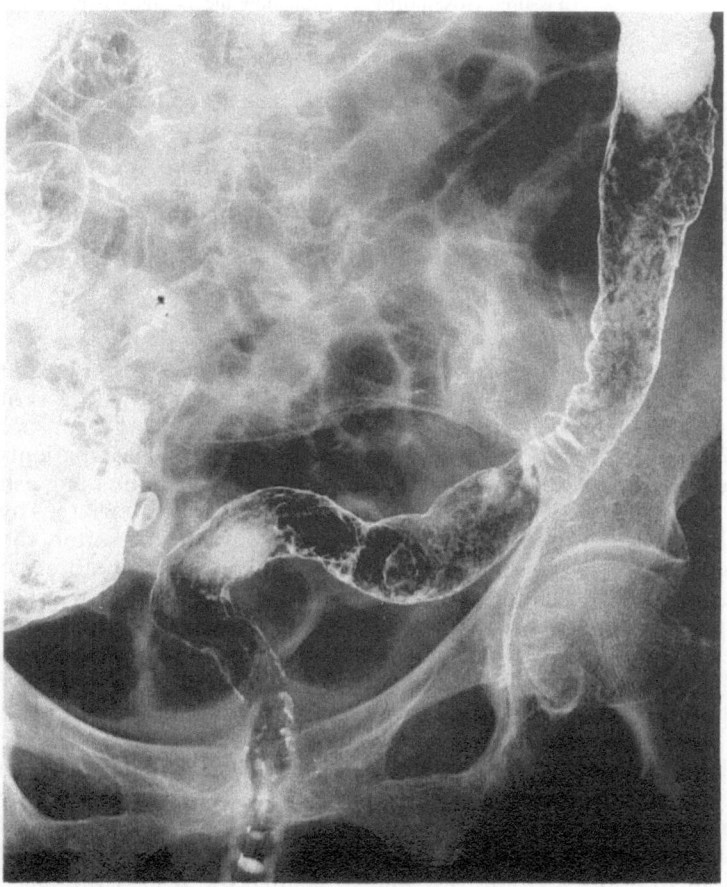

Fig. 7.5. Air contrast barium enema showing ulcerative colitis of distal large bowel.

Table 7.1. Diagnosis of Crohn's disease and ulcerative colitis

	Crohn's disease	Ulcerative colitis
Clinical features		
Abdominal pain	+ve	−ve
Abdominal mass	+ve (50%)	−ve
Rectal bleeding	Rarely	+ve
Fistula formation	+ve (5–8%)	+ve (2–3%)
Perianal suppuration	+ve (40%)	+ve (15%)
Rectal involvement	+ve (40%)	+ve (95%)
Carcinoma	Rare (3–5%)	+ve (15% after 15 years)
Radiology		
Rectum	−ve	+ve
Small bowel	+ve (skip lesions)	Rare (18% reflux ileitis)
Strictures	+ve	Very rare
Mucosa	Fissures (rosethorn)	Shallow ulcers and polyps
Histology	Sarcoid granulomas in 70%	Non-specific inflammation

the creation of a permanent ileal stoma (ileostomy) or an ileoanal anastomosis with formation of an ileal pouch.

Stoma Management

The end result of many of the procedures described in this section is that the patient is left not only with a large abdominal scar but also with a vent in the abdominal wall through which intestinal contents discharge and are collected in disposable plastic bags. Not surprisingly, many of these patients have mental as well as physical scars to contend with. The patient's anguish at having to live with a permanent stoma can be greatly alleviated by arranging visits from a voluntary support group before and after the operation. Preoperative counselling gives the patient confidence before the operation and, after discharge from hospital, membership of one or other of these groups allows the patient to be informed of recent developments in stoma care. The patient also benefits from regular contact with others who have had personal experience of living with an ileostomy or colostomy.

The stomatherapist has an important role in management of the abdominal conduit. The therapist is hospital-based and conducts outpatient clinics but is also available for domiciliary visits to stoma patients. Diversity in the shape and contour of the patient's abdominal wall makes siting of the ostomy important. The site of choice for the stoma will therefore be clearly marked on the abdominal wall before operation. Postoperatively the therapist will teach the patient to apply a stoma ring and to change the disposable bags. Adequate care and hygiene of the stoma itself and of the surrounding skin are of paramount importance for the patient's comfort and wellbeing. The stomatherapist is an integral part of the surgical team caring for patients who have to live with a permanent abdominal stoma.

Spasmodic Intestinal Disorders Producing Pelvic Pain

Proctalgia Fugax

In this uncommon disorder the patient experiences a sudden acute pain in the rectum, lasting 2 to 3 minutes and relieved by the passing of flatus. The rectal pain is due to overdistension of the rectum by flatus, with spasm of both the rectosigmoid junction and the external sphincter muscles. Proctalgia is not associated with any intrinsic bowel disease. Relief from the rectal pain occurs spontaneously, but the patient can be taught to relieve the pain quickly by self-dilatation of the anal canal to release flatus.

Irritable Bowel Syndrome

In this syndrome persistent, colicky lower abdominal pain is associated with anorexia, belching, abdominal distension and the passage of small, hard faecal boluses. Occasionally the patient will have bouts of mucoid diarrhoea alternating with constipation. The symptoms are produced by excessive colonic motility and spasm of the bowel (spastic colon) and in many cases the disorder has a large psychogenic component. As the symptoms of this syndrome are similar to those of diverticular disease or a colonic neoplasm, the patient will need to be fully investigated for these conditions before a diagnosis of spastic colon is made. A barium enema may demonstrate narrowing and segmentation of the pelvic colon.

Treatment is often ineffective. Anticholinergic, antispasmodic drugs, such as Buscopan, may be helpful in some patients.

Neoplasms of the Large Bowel

Benign Adenomas of the Rectum and Sigmoid Colon

Adenomas are the commonest benign tumours of the large bowel, and two types are encountered: simple adenoma and villous adenoma.

Simple Adenoma. A simple adenoma is often encountered in infancy and childhood and presents with rectal bleeding. A juvenile adenoma becomes pedunculated and frequently prolapses through the anus. This type of adenoma never becomes malignant. Treatment is surgical excision. Simple sessile adenomas in adults may be multiple, and 80 % are found in the rectum and sigmoid colon. If larger than 1 cm the adenoma should be endoscopically excised and sent for histological examination, since 5 % will

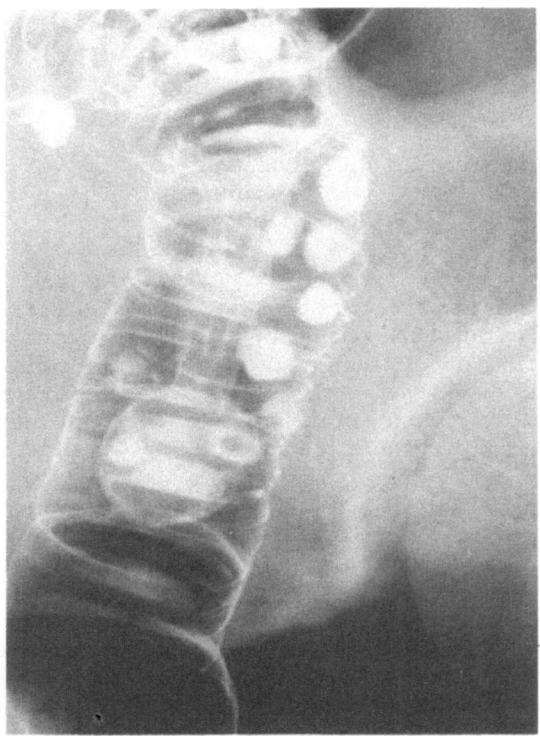

Fig. 7.6. Barium enema showing a pedunculated rectosigmoid polyp and sigmoid diverticula.

show evidence of malignant change. Benign polyps in the rectum are frequently asymptomatic, but rectal bleeding and prolapse through the anus may occur, with occasionally some discomfort in the lower rectum. Larger rectosigmoid pedunculated polyps may (Fig. 7.6) produce an intussusception through the anal orifice and cause the patient considerable discomfort and pain. Patients with multiple rectosigmoid adenomas should be kept under annual surveillance with a sigmoidoscopy and colonoscopy, since in 5 % of patients these polyps undergo malignant transformation.

Villous Ademoma. This tumour accounts for 10 % of adenomas in the large bowel, and the majority (up to 80 %) are found in the rectum and sigmoid colon. A villous adenoma is a premalignant condition, and 30 % of untreated tumours will become malignant. The lesion is broad based, shaggy and fronded and will probably occupy a large area of the wall of the large bowel. The villi of the adenoma secrete large quantitites of potassium-laden mucin. Clinically the lesion is painless and rarely bleeds. Bleeding from a villous adenoma nearly always indicates malignant transformation.

Diagnosis is made with rectal finger examination and sigmoidoscopy. Treatment is by transrectal excision provided the patient is young and fit enough for surgery. Large lesions and premalignant villous adenomata will need an abdominoperineal resection of the rectum for complete eradication.

Malignant Tumours of the Large Bowel

Seventy per cent of carcinomas of the large bowel are located in the rectum and sigmoid colon and 10 % in the caecum. The remaining large-bowel carcinomas are distributed throughout the ascending, transverse and descending colon. More than 17 000 people a year in the United Kingdom die of a cancer of the colon or rectum, with an equal sex distribution. Known aetiological factors are: familial polyposis (cancer develops at about 25 years of age), colonic adenomas or polyps (5 % are malignant), villous adenoma (30 % of untreated tumours become malignant) and ulcerative colitis (15 % incidence of malignancy after 15 years). Seventy-five per cent of all these conditions occur in the rectosigmoid segment of the large bowel. Stasis of faecal carcinogens in the rectosigmoid area has been postulated as an aetiological factor. Four pathological types of tumour are possible: polypoidal; ulcerative; annular; and proliferative. Most tumours start as polypoidal lesions and subsequently ulcerate or proliferate. Proliferative and ulcerative lesions are commoner in the capacious rectum and caecum. An annular carcinoma is commoner in the sigmoid colon, where constriction leads to intestinal obstruction. Polypoidal and proliferative lesions in the rectosigmoid junction may protrude into the rectum as an intussuseption with features of intermittent intestinal obstruction. Histologically the lesion is an adenocarcinoma, with evidence of mucoid degeneration in 10 %. Colonic and rectal tumours spread locally, by the lymphatics or by the bloodstream. Extension through the bowel wall may fix the tumour to the musculoskeletal walls of the pelvic cavity or to surrounding organs and may produce fistulae into the small intestine (coloenteric), bladder (colovesical) or vagina (rectovaginal). Advanced rectal tumours are frequently "fixed" to the sacral hollow. Lymphatic spread is to local nodes (pararectal and paracolic) and then along the inferior mesenteric vessels to the mesenteric lymph nodes. Bloodstream spread (portal) is mainly to the liver, but metastases may occur in the lungs and brain. Duke's pathological staging of resected rectal tumour uses the degree of spread to the lymph nodes as an indication of prognosis and as an evaluation of the various treatments used in the management of colorectal tumours (Table 7.2). The overall survival rate for all cases of colorectal carcinoma is between 20 % and 30 %. In 15 % of patients a second primary (metachranous) tumour will be present elsewhere in the large bowel.

All carcinomas of the terminal large bowel are accessible either by digital examination of the rectum or by sigmoidoscopy and colonoscopy for growths above the rectosigmoid junction. The patient with a rectal growth complains of bleeding piles or rectal bleeding with alteration of bowel habit, urgency, passage of mucus, tenesmus and a feeling of incomplete emptying of the

Table 7.2. Duke's staging of resected rectal tumour

Stage	5 year survival (%)
A. Confined to mucosa	95
B. Involving muscle	80
C1. Local nodes involved	50
C2. Involved nodes at pelvic brim	40
C3. Inferior mesenteric nodes involved	30

bowel. Pain is not a prominent complaint, but tenesmus may be troublesome, and deep pain within the pelvis is a poor prognostic sign, since it may indicate spread of the tumour into the sacral nerve plexuses or the anal canal.

A patient with a carcinoma of the sigmoid colon will have the above features with superadded bouts of colicky abdominal pain and "explosive" diarrhoea, when he or she will experience sharp lower abdominal pains and urgency to defaecate. However, at stool the patient passes only flatus and a bloody mucoid diarrhoea. In 50 % of patients abdominal examination reveals a mass in the left iliac fossa, due either to faecal impaction behind the tumour or to the tumour itself.

Routine examination must include an examination of the upper abdomen for signs of metastatic hepatomegaly. Nearly all rectal growths can be diagnosed with the index finger when the ulcerating or proliferative tumour will be palpable. Digital examination of the upper rectum may be aided by asking the patient to strain gently against the examining finger. Sigmoidoscopic examination will visualise the tumour, and multiple biopsy specimens can be obtained. Colonoscopy may be necessary for a complete examination of the sigmoid colon. A barium enema examination is complementary to endoscopy and will demonstrate a colonic carcinoma but not necessarily a rectal tumour. Radiology will also exclude a metachronous tumour in the large bowel.

Ten per cent of annular carcinomas obstruct the bowel, and these are treated by means of a temporary transverse colostomy followed 3 to 4 weeks later by definitive resection and closure of the colostomy. Carcinomas of the sigmoid colon, the rectosigmoid junction and upper half of the rectum are treated by anterior resection with complete excision of the lymphatic field of drainage. A carcinoma of the distal half of the rectum is treated with rectal excision and formation of a permanent left iliac colostomy. Some patients with small tumours of the distal rectum may be treated by endoanal local excision and preservation of the anal sphincter. Irresectable tumours of the rectum remain a problem as they are not radiosensitive and respond poorly to chemotherapy.

The caecum is the site for a carcinoma in 10 % of patients with large-bowel cancer in the 40 to 70 age group. Caecal carcinoma is commoner in women than men.

Symptoms are vague dyspepsia, malaise, lassitude, weight loss and diarrhoea. Secondary anaemia is also common. Half the patients have a palpable mass in the right iliac fossa. About 20 % of patients present with intestinal obstruction. Investigation of an unexplained secondary hypochromic anaemia in an elderly woman must include a barium enema examination, which may demonstrate a filling defect in the caecum. An appendix abscess, Crohn's disease or a right ovarian tumour or cyst are differential diagnoses of a caecal neoplasm.

Resectable tumours of the caecum are treated by means of a right hemicolectomy. Irresectable tumours are treated with a palliative ileo-transverse anastomosis.

Metastatic and Recurrent Tumours

The female pelvis is a depository for malignant tissue in one of four circumstances:

Incomplete removal of a primary carcinoma within the pelvis

Recurrence after surgical resection or radiotherapy treatment of a pelvic neoplasm

Metastatic deposits from a primary lesion elsewhere in the abdominal cavity

Pelvic deposits in malignant ascites, especially ovarian secondary tumour.

The commonest carcinomas which produce a "pelvic recurrence" are those of the ovary, cervix, rectum and bladder. Whatever the source of the primary tumour, recurrent disease will involve the pelvic organs and may eventually infiltrate the sacral plexuses and lateral pelvic walls, producing severe somatic pelvic pain. In some instances the recurrent tumour may infiltrate into the perineum or vagina, producing somatic perineal pain. The intrapelvic ureters are in jeopardy, and obstruction of one or other, and sometimes both, is common. The pain caused by pelvic recurrent disease is often severe and intractable.

A few patients, in whom recurrence is confined to the remaining viscera in the pelvis, may be suitable for a pelvic exenteration. In these circumstances the patients will have a permanent iliac colostomy and an ileal conduit for urinary diversion. In the majority of patients the recurrent tumour will not be amenable to further surgery, and radiotherapy or chemotherapy may be effective symptomatic palliation. In the presence of intractable pain phenol blocks of the somatic and perineal nerves may be the only palliative therapy possible.

Differential Diagnosis of Palpable Tumours of the Greater Pelvis

Palpable masses in the lower abdomen, below the umbilicus, can present difficulties in diagnosis. The abdominal component of the greater pelvis is conveniently divided into three regions: right and left iliac and hypogastric. The differential diagnosis of masses palpated in this region is depicted in Tables 7.3, 7.4 and 7.5.

Table 7.3. Palpable tumours of the greater pelvis: hypogastrium

Pain	Discomfort
Acute retention of urine	Chronic retention of urine
Torsion or haemorrhage into right or left ovarian cyst	Haematocolpos (childhood)
Haematometra	Gravid uterus
	Fibroid uterus
	Large right or left ovarian cyst or carcinoma
	Carcinoma or sarcoma of uterus

Table 7.4. Palpable tumours of the greater pelvis: right iliac fossa

Pain	Discomfort
Appendix mass	Right ovarian cyst or carcinoma
Ileocaecal Crohn's disease	Carcinoma of caecum
Torsion right ovarian cyst	Mesenteric cyst
	Meckel's diverticulum
	Right pelvic ectopic kidney

Table 7.5. Palpable tumours of the greater pelvis: left iliac fossa

Pain	Discomfort
Diverticular abscess	Carcinoma of sigmoid colon
Torsion left ovarian cyst	Diverticular mass
	Left ovarian cyst or carcinoma
	Left pelvic ectopic kidney

Vascular Disorders Producing Pelvic Pain

Aortoiliac Embolism and Thrombosis

The iliac arteries may be gradually occluded by atherosclerosis or obstructed by an embolus. The resultant ischaemia produces pain in the affected limb but may also give rise to pelvic pain. Aortoiliac occlusion in normotensive women between 35 and 55 years of age occurs in those with very narrow iliac vessels. (Fig. 7.7).

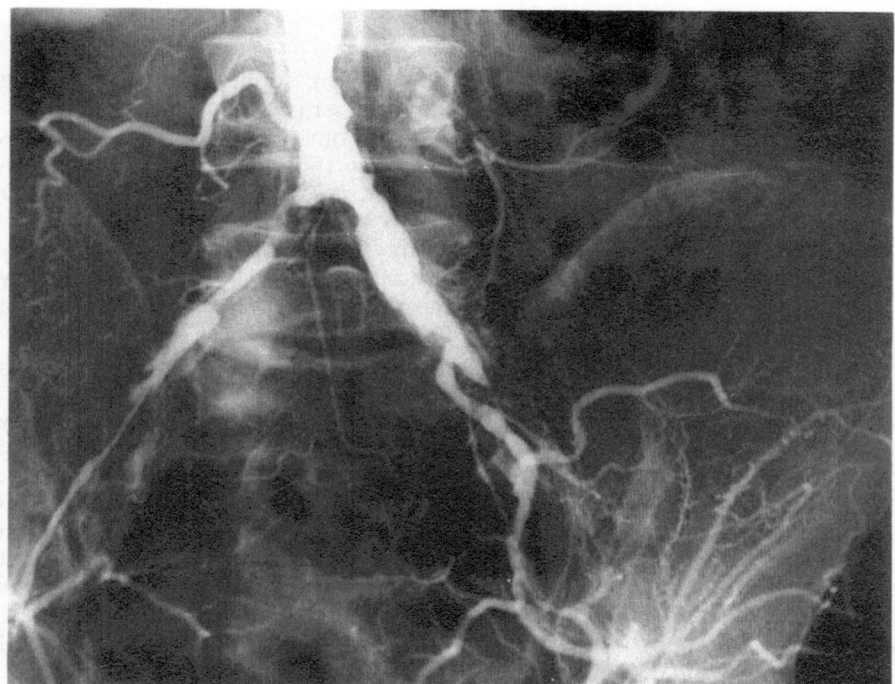

Fig. 7.7. Arteriogram showing widespread atheroma with occlusion of left external iliac artery and collateral circulation.

Whether the occlusion is thrombotic or embolic, the patient will complain of pain in the affected limb and probably pain in the buttocks. The pain is characteristically aggravated by exercise (claudication). The affected limb becomes colder and paler, and in sudden occlusion diminished sensation to pinprick may be demonstrated.

Routine clinical examination of a woman with chronic pelvic and buttock pain includes palpation of the femoral and distal arteries for pulsation and auscultation of the iliofemoral areas for a bruit. Absence of femoral and distal pulses and a bruit over a partially occluded iliac vessel are characteristic signs of aortoiliac occlusion. Investigations for aortoiliac occlusion include a Döppler ultrasound detector and venous occlusion plethysmography (in which the size of the limb is measured after occluding venous outflow; in occlusive disease diminished venous return induces restriction of arterial inflow). Femoral arteriography will demonstate the occlusion site.

Acute obstruction to the iliac arteries by an embolus is an acute surgical emergency and should be treated by means of urgent embolectomy. Chronic symptomatic aortoiliac atherosclerosis is treated by excision of the occluded vessels and the insertion of an aortoiliac graft.

Iliac Vein Thrombosis

Thrombosis of the large iliac veins may occur spontaneously, following injury to the lower limb and pelvis or appear after pelvic surgical procedures. An estimated 30 % of patients have asymptomatic deep vein thrombosis after major surgery. Thrombosis occluding the iliac vein produces an enlarged, warm and painful leg. The patient rarely experiences pain or discomfort in the pelvis. In a proportion of patients the thrombosis lies loosely attached to the vein wall and may break away and be carried by the venous flow to the lungs. In 20 % of patients who suffer pulmonary emboli the source of the embolus is the pelvic vein. The cardinal causes of venous thrombosis (Virchow's triad) are stasis, changes in thrombogenicity of the blood and changes in the vessel wall. Venous stasis may occur during prolonged immobilisation or after major surgery or injury. External pressure on the vein from enlarged lymph nodes, tumours or during pregnancy may lead to venous thrombosis. High-dose oestrogen oral contraceptives in the young and cancer in older women may be predisposing thrombolytic agents.

Diagnosis is made from the presenting symptoms of leg pain with enlargement and dependent oedema and it may initially be impossible until a complication such as pulmonary embolism occurs. In the group with silent thrombosis clinical examination is seldom rewarding. Venography remains the standard method for detecting thrombi in the larger vessels. Isotope screening, Döppler scanning and impedance plethysmography may be helpful in further investigation.

The mainstay of management in the majority of patients is prevention combined with anticoagulant therapy. During anaesthesia the pumping action of the leg muscles is maintained by ensheathing the lower limbs in stockings which are intermittently inflated and by administration of therapeutic doses of mini-heparin. Elasticated stockings are worn for a further week, and early ambulation is encouraged. Established venous thrombosis is treated with intravenous heparin (heparin pump) for the first week and subsequently with oral anticoagulants (Phenisidione 75–100 mg daily) continued for at least six weeks, the dose being carefully monitored by means of the coagulation time. Surgical removal of the clot from the pelvic veins and partial occlusion of the vena cava to prevent a pulmonary embolus migrating centrally are not widely used in the management of these patients.

Orthopaedic Causes of Pelvic Pain

D.G. Jones

In general, orthopaedic causes of pelvic pain in the female are easily recognised by their distribution and quality. They are usually made worse by exercise and weight bearing and relieved by rest. Physical signs of joint or locomotive disorder are usually present.

Posterior Pelvic Pain

Pain Originating in the Lumbosacral Spine

This usually presents with localised pain in the lower lumbar spine and over the sacrum, often radiating over the sacroiliac ligaments and referred into the posterior thigh and buttock. Should there be referred pain in the true sciatic distribution and in the S1 or L5 nerve roots then pain is felt below the knee joint. This may be accompanied by signs of nerve root disorder, such as dermatome sensory deficit or myotome weakness. In elderly patients neurogenic claudication is not uncommon. This is usually related to increasing discomfort in the buttock or thigh, less frequently in the calf following exercise. It can be differentiated from vascular claudication in that the exercise tolerance is greater and relief following resting of pain takes considerably longer. It is also evident on examining the patient following exercise when significant signs of nerve root dysfunction might present.

Treatment is based on the general treatment of lumbar problems, and rest may be all that is required to relieve the symptoms. However, more definitive treatment in the form of traction and manipulative therapy may be useful. Lumbar disc surgery is rarely considered for the relief of postural pelvic pain and is more likely to be reserved for nerve root entrapment with more distal signs and symptoms.

Sacroiliac Joint Pain

Disorders of the sacroiliac joint are usually related to inflammatory arthritis of the ankylosing spondylitis variety. This is not, as previously thought, rare in women but is less common than in men. Pain radiating from the sacroiliac joint can commonly be felt in both the buttock and the posterior thigh and is often aggravated by rotation of the lumbar spine on the pelvis. There is usually discomfort over the diseased sacroiliac joint, and the pain is made worse by weight bearing. The other major cause of chronic sacroiliac pain is trauma. The sacroiliac ligaments are probably the strongest ligaments in the body, and disruption of these demands massive high-velocity trauma. If this is the case then long-term morbidity is likely, because the sacroiliac joint commonly becomes osteoarthritic. The "subluxated" sacroiliac joint which is commonly diagnosed as a cause of lower lumbar or posterior pelvic pain is a misnomer. The strength of the ligaments surrounding this joint is such that minor subluxation unrelated to massive trauma is impossible.

In ankylosing spondylitis the principles of management are clear and based on the continuing need to maintain mobility, along with analgesic and anti-inflammatory medication. In established osteoarthritis following trauma surgical fusion may occasionally be helpful.

Coccydynia and Sacrococcygeal Pain

This is a very common presentation in women. It is often associated with a fall on to the buttocks and presents with difficulty in sitting on firm surfaces and pain in the coccygeal region on defaecation or straining. The coccyx is very tender on palpation, particularly per rectum.

Treatment is usually in the form of hydrocortisone injection, and occasionally manipulation of the coccyx may be required. In rare circumstances coccygectomy is indicated if the pain is intractable, but this is rarely successful if the coccydynia is associated with more diffuse lumbosacral pain.

Proximal Hamstring Injury (Including Avulsion of the Ischial Epiphysis in the Adolescent)

In the physically active patient this is a common cause of posterior pelvic and buttock pain and can be extremely severe in the adolescent when the ischial tuberosity is avulsed. This may present with a gross bony overgrowth and an X-ray picture suggestive of a primary bone tumour. This latter appearance is due to the excessive periosteal reaction related to the separation of the epiphysis.

Treatment is by rest and local physiotherapy.

Superficial Abscesses Including Pilonidal Abscess

Abscesses of the post-natal cleft are common in the form of a pilonidal disorder. A pilonidal sinus is an abnormal tract in the postnatal cleft lined with epithelium and in many cases containing hair. It is rare in women. Most pilonidal sinuses develop in adult life between 20 and 30 years of age and, in the absence of sepsis, are symptomless. A typical sinus will be evident as a small, often pustular opening about 2 cm posterior to the anus. The opening leads to a tract which can extend headwards in the subcutaneous tissue for up to 5 cm. Lateral extension may occur into the buttocks, as also may further midline openings in the skin of the post-natal cleft. The main complication of a pilonidal sinus is sepsis, which occurs in most patients at some stage and leads to the formation of a pilonidal abscess, appearing as a tender painful lump, subsequently with purulent bloody discharge.

The condition has to be differentiated from a perianal abscess or acute bone pain in the lower sacrum and coccyx.

Surgical drainage relieves the acute pain. When the inflammation has subsided formal excision and primary suturing are performed. There is a high incidence of recurrence following primary suturing, and in these cases the cavity after excision of the abscess is left to granulate. Some surgeons advocate the use of a silastic bung to aid healing of the chronically infected cavity.

Anterior Pelvic Problems

Hip Joint (Fig. 7.8)

The hip joint is supplied mainly by branches of the obturator and femoral nerves and pain related to any disorder of this joint can therefore commonly

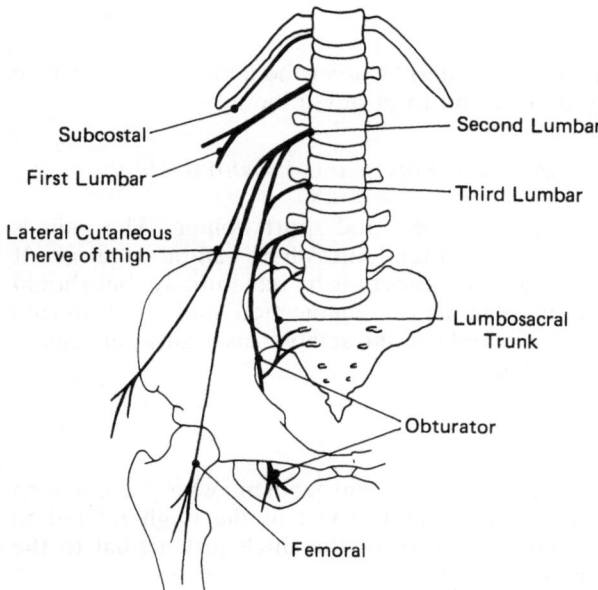

Fig. 7.8. Root origin of lateral cutaneous nerve of thigh, obturator nerve and femoral nerve.

be referred along the distribution of these nerves. Hip joint pain is most commonly felt in the groin and the anterior thigh and often can be radiated medially down the thigh as far as the knee via the obturator nerve (Fig. 7.8).

Treatment depends on the exact cause of hip joint disease. Inflammatory arthritis can be treated medically with anti-inflammatory drugs, but once joint destruction takes place then total joint replacement is the only effective remedy.

Symphysis Pubis

In the pregnant woman separation of the symphysis pubis before parturition can be quite alarming as a presentation clinically. Separation normally resolves following birth of the child and requires no active treatment. The chronic symphysitis pubis usually responds to rest and local physiotherapy, but rarely a fusion of the symphysis pubis may be indicated for intractable cases.

Local Injury to the Insertion of the Rectus Abdominis

This is not uncommon in athletic individuals and merely presents with either a haematoma or localised pain and tenderness over the insertion of the rectus abdominis. Treatment is by rest, local steroid injection and physiotherapy.

Rectus Femoris Insertion Injuries

This presents as localised pain and tenderness over the anterior inferior iliac spine. Treatment is mainly by rest and local physiotherapy.

Pain in the Adductor Region of the Pelvis and Proximal Thigh

This is a common presentation in dancers and sportswomen. The pain is localised to the adductor insertion, and tenderness here can be exquisite. It is aggravated by resisted adduction. Treatment is by rest initially, but should the pain not settle then anti-inflammatory medication and local steroid injection may be required. Very rarely in intractable cases surgical release of the adductor origin may be indicated.

Neuralgia Paraesthetica

This condition is often seen in obese or gravid women, who present with paraesthesiae and discomfort in the lateral aspect of the thigh related to entrapment of the lateral cutaneous nerve of the thigh just medial to the anterior superior iliac spine (Fig. 7.8.).

Symptoms are often relieved by weight loss, but occasionally injection locally around the nerve or surgical release may be indicated.

Femoral Neuralgia

In more proximal lumbar disc lesions (L 2/3 or 3/4) the femoral nerve roots can be affected, and pain radiates into the corresponding dermatomes. There is usually accompanying lumbar backache and lumbar muscle spasm. There can be signs of weakness of the quadriceps and numbness in the affected dermatome. A positive femoral stretch test can be elicited, with the patient prone, by extending the hip with the ipsilateral knee flexed. Excruciating pain in the anterior thigh prevents further extension of the hip.

As in the sciatic nerve root irritation, rest is usually all that is required, although should the pain be intractable and not settle with rest and inpatient traction, further investigations including lumbar myelography or computed tomography may be indicated as a preoperative aid. Local disc excision can then be performed to relieve the nerve root irritation.

Psoas Abscess

This presents with swelling and discomfort in the groin, with the hip held flexed and adducted. It is associated with tuberculosis or pyogenic lumbar vertebral infections and is now very rarely seen. Treatment depends on the cause and should be directed toward the focus of infection in the lumbar spine. In tuberculosis chemotherapy is usually all that is required.

Generalised Diseases Affecting the Pelvis

The bones of the pelvis as well as the joints can be affected by generalised diseases, including infection and tumour, as well as more specific diseases of bone such as Paget's disease.

Infection

Osteomyelitis can occur acutely in any of the areas of the pelvis and presents with the usual picture of generalised malaise and pyrexia with localised severe pain and tenderness. Treatment is usually with chemotherapy (for 6 weeks), but occasionally surgical drainage may be required. The offending organism is usually a staphylococcus. Chronic infection can be related to inadequately treated acute osteomyelitis and also to tuberculosis.

Septic Arthritis of the Sacroiliac Joint

This is exceedingly rare and usually results in severe degenerative change within the joint, which may in some cases require surgical fusion. Septic arthritis of the hip in the adult is uncommon and must be treated vigorously with arthrotomy and drainage as well as chemotherapy if the likely sequelae of osteoarthrosis is to be avoided.

Tumours of Bone

Secondary carcinomas are by far the most common tumours of the bony pelvis, the most common primary sites being breast, lung, thyroid, and kidney. Primary tumours of the pelvis are rare, the most likely being a chondrosarcoma in a middle-aged patient. Lymphoma affecting bone can be seen in the pelvic bones also.

Treatment of tumours of bone are obviously specific to the individual tumour or to the primary carcinoma in secondary bone tumours. Because of the anatomy of the pelvis with its closely associated neurovascular structures, radiotherapy is often preferred to surgical excision.

Metabolic Disorders of Bone

Stress fractures of the pubis are not uncommon in osteomalacia and in Paget's disease. Occasionally local biopsy may be required to exclude secondary tumour. Paget's disease of bone frequently affects the pelvis but is generally painless unless it secondarily affects the joints by causing osteoarthrosis or stress fractures or very rarely when malignant change occurs in the Paget's disease.

Management clearly depends on the diagnosis. Both osteomalacia and Paget's disease can be treated with chemotherapy, although surgical intervention may be required for secondary osteoarthrosis of joints. Pelvic pain in the female is frequently caused by orthopaedic disorders. It is invariably made worse by exercise and commonly relieved by rest. It is usually associated with physical signs related to the particular joint or part of the pelvic wall involved.

8 Pain Management

G.D. THOMAS

It is most important to appreciate the difference between the treatment requirements of acute as opposed to chronic or intractable pain.

By definition, acute pain is of sudden onset and usually of limited duration. It is often intermittent, and treatment of the pain takes place in parallel with other measures designed to diagnose and specifically treat its cause. The pain serves a useful purpose in alerting the patient and physician that something is wrong.

Intractable pain, on the other hand, particularly when associated with malignancy, no longer serves a useful purpose – on the contrary it leads to decreasing mobility and increasing reliance on supportive relatives, nursing and medical staff. It is constant and tends to get worse with time. The patient's reaction to this type of pain is vastly different to that induced by acute pain; the most careful attention to analgesia will be of paramount importance.

The basic principle of prescribing for any type of pain is that the potency and dosage should be the minimum required to produce the desired level of analgesia so that side-effects will be minimised. In acute pain, which is usually intermittent, prescribing on an "as required" basis is acceptable. In chronic pain constant 24 hour control must be aimed at, so the drugs must be given at regular intervals. Knowledge of the duration of action of drugs is therefore imperative.

For convenience, pain is usually categorised as mild, moderate or severe.

Mild Pain

For mild pain the drugs of choice are aspirin, paracetamol and non-steroidal anti-inflammatory drugs (NSAIDs) (Table 8.1).

Aspirin has a useful anti-inflammatory effect because of its antiprostaglandin properties. However, a common side-effect is gastric intolerance.

Table 8.1. Drugs for the treatment of mild pain

Drug	Dose	Duration of action	Comments
Aspirin	300–600 mg	4 hours	Anti-inflammatory. Gastric intolerance fairly common
Paracetamol	0.5–1.0 g	4 hours	No anti-inflammatory activity. May cause liver damage in overdosage. Generally well tolerated
Non-steroidal anti-inflammatory drugs		6–24 hours	See below

Caution: Age, peptic ulceration, allergy (asthma), pregnancy, renal and hepatic insufficiency, drug interactions.

Paracetomol has no anti-inflammatory activity but may cause liver damage in high dosage. It is generally well tolerated.

Like aspirin, NSAIDs have anti-prostaglandin activity and are effective in inflammatory disorders. They are particularly effective in musculoskeletal disorders, including malignant secondary skeletal metastases. They are also useful in dysmenorrhoea. The anti-inflammatory activity of NSAIDs varies from drug to drug, as does the frequency of side-effects. Patient response is very variable, sos it is always prudent to start treatment with a low dose of one of the less potent NSAIDs, such as ibuprofen, and gradually increase dosage or potency as required.

Moderate Pain

Codeine, dihydrocodeine and dextropropoxyphene, the three drugs most commonly used in moderate pain, are weak narcotics and as such may be addictive. While this presents no problem when prescribed for early malignant pain, in chronic benign pain this potential should be carefully considered. All three are often prescribed in combination with aspirin or paracetamol in lower dosage. The combination of paracetamol and dextropropoxyphene (Co-proxamol) may provide effective analgesia for mild to moderate pain. A disadvantage of Co-proxamol is that overdosage may lead to respiratory depression and hepatotoxicity.

Table 8.2. Drugs used for the treatment of moderate pain

Drug	Dose	Duration of action	Comments
Codeine	30–60 mg	4 hours	Available as tablets, syrup or injection. Generally well tolerated but constipating
Dihydro-codeine (DHC)	30–60 mg	4 hours	May cause dizziness in ambulatory patients. Constipating. Available as tablets syrup or injection
DHC continus	60 mg	12 hours	Sustained release tablet available
Dextroprop-oxyphene	65 mg	6 hours	May cause sedation and dizziness. Constipating

Severe Pain

Severe pain requires more potent drugs. The weak narcotics mentioned above have a ceiling effect, so increasing their dosage is not effective.

Acute Pain

Severe acute pain requires prompt treatment, and this usually means intramuscular or intravenous injection. Morphine is the classic strong opiate and remains the standard against which all others are compared. Characteristics of morphine and related opiates are shown in Table 8.3. Of the side-effects, respiratory depression is potentially the most harmful, but in clinical practice it should rarely be a problem if the dosage is related carefully to the patient's age, body weight and general condition. Patients with pre-existing respiratory disease tolerate morphine least well, and the drug is contraindicated in conditions where a rise in PCO_2 is undesirable (e.g. head injuries). Drugs (other than morphine) used in the treatment of severe pain are shown in Table 8.4.

The classic opiates are pure agonists, and their actions can be reversed specifically by naloxone. Some analgesics have antagonist activity, i.e. they interfere with the actions of agonists while producing analgesia at other receptor sites; an example is pentazocine. Buprenorphine, another potent analgesic, exhibits partial agonist activity, and in high dosage it may even oppose the effect of agonists. Buprenorphine analgesia is slow in onset but lasts 6 to 8 hours. The drug is effectively absorbed sublingually, but it commonly causes nausea and vomiting (but this may be controlled by antiemetics) and occasionally dizziness, sweating and oversedation. Its effects are only partially reversed by naloxone. There is a ceiling analgesic effect, so exceeding the usual dose is rarely indicated. The usual dose for severe pain is 0.3 mg by injection or 0.4 mg sublingually.

Table 8.3. Characteristics of morphine and related opiates

Desirable features	Side effects
Strong analgesia	Respiratory depression
Good anxiolysis	Nausea and/or vomiting
Sedation	Constipation
	Addictive potential

Table 8.4. Some other strong analgesics

Drug	Duration	IM dose equivalent to morphine 10 mg	Comments
Papaveretum	4 hours	15 mg	Contains all opium alkaloids including 50% morphine
Diamorphine	4 hours	5 mg	Euphoriant. Possibly less nauseating and constipating than morphine
Pethidine	3 hours	75 mg	Minimal anxiolysis. Good antispasmodic. Better for visceral than somatic pain

Chronic Pain

Benign Chronic Pain

Chronic pain in non-malignant conditions can be severe and not controllable by the analgesics used for mild to moderate pain. However, in patients with non-malignant conditions it is important to avoid the use of opiates because of their addiction potential.

Depression is a common accompaniment of chronic pain states and, whether the depression is of primary or secondary aetiology, treatment with an antidepressant should always be considered. The tricyclic antidepressants seem to have analgesia enhancing properties – the pain of postherpetic neuralgia, for instance, has been shown to be reduced by amitriptyline.

Where pain is thought to be secondary to nerve damage or neuropathy, an anticonvulsant is indicated, e.g. sodium valproate 100 – 200 mg tds.

If the patient does not come under the above categories and careful psychological assessment does not indicate a supratentorial reason for the pain, then the following drugs may be considered because of their low addiction potential:

1. Buprenorphine 0.2–0.4 mg sublingually 8 hourly.
2. Pentazocine 50–100 mg orally 4 hourly. Being an antagonist-type analgesic, pentazocine may precipitate withdrawal symptoms in patients

previously dependent on narcotic analgesics. Occasionally dysphoria including hallucinations may occur.

3. Meptazinol and Nalbuphine are analgesics that may find a place in the treatment of severe chronic benign pain, although Nalbuphine is available only as an injection at present.

Although these drugs have a lower addiction potential than the classic opiates, patients may become dependent on them and they are best reserved for short periods to treat exacerbations of pain.

Chronic Pain of Malignancy

Treatment of the severe pain of malignancy requires strong opiates in adequate dosage at regular intervals. Whenever possible, medication should be given orally.

Morphine is the drug most often used and is best titrated as an oral solution 4 hourly until adequate control is achieved. At this time the patient may be transferred to the same total dose given as MST continus tablets 12 hourly. Nausea, if encountered, can be relieved with an antiemetic such as prochlorperazine or haloperidol, but nausea caused by morphine rarely lasts longer than a week. Respiratory depression is never seen if the drug is titrated carefully up to its effective dose. Severe pain is a very good antagonist of opiate induced respiratory depression. Oversedation can be an early problem but usually lessens with time. Constipation is an invariable result of opiate medication and requires aperients and dietary advice (if appropriate). If oral medication is not possible (e.g. because of intractable vomiting) then parenteral administration must be considered. This is best achieved by using a constant subcutaneous infusion of diamorphine. Diamorphine is preferred for this route of administration because of its high solubility in water. The total daily oral dose of morphine should be divided by three to arrive at the equivalent dose of diamorphine required by injection per day.

Alternatives to morphine for the control of severe pain of malignancy are shown in Table 8.5.

There are a number of drugs which will contribute to pain relief in specific situations. In *bone pain* non-steroidal anti-inflammatory drugs, by inhibiting prostaglandin synthetase at the site of bony malignancy, considerably enhance opioid analgesia. When an expanding pelvic tumour causes *nerve compression* (involving the sacral nerves or nerve roots), a corticosteroid is indicated to relieve surrounding inflammation and oedema. Dexamethasone in a dosage of 4 to 16 mg daily is effective. For nerve root irritation causing severe lancinating pains an anticonvulsant such as sodium valproate 200 mg tid is helpful. For *muscle spasms* a small dose of diazepam 2 mg tds, increasing as necessary, is often helpful. For more resistant cases baclofen 5 mg tds, increasing if necessary, is a more powerful choice but may cause undesirable hypotonia. *Sphincter spasms* can be distressing and can often be relieved with chlorpromazine.

Table 8.5. Alternatives to oral morphine

Drug		Dose interval	Remarks	Equivalent dose of oral morphine
Levorphanol	1.5 mg	8 hours	Less sedating	10 mg
Phenazocine	2.5 mg	6 hours	Less sedating. Does not contract sphincter of Oddi. Absorbed sublingually	12.5 mg
Oxycodone	30 mg	8 hours	Useful alternative to oral therapy	15 mg
Dextromoramide	5 mg	2 hours	Useful for breakthrough pain only	15 mg

When planning analgesia for a patient with malignant disease, the precise reason for every pain complained of should be sought and treated as specifically as possible. If the patient remains oversedated during the daytime by the minimum effective analgesic dose of morphine, then it is reasonable to substitute one of the less sedating opiates. This can then be combined with a substantial evening dose of morphine to ensure a good night's sleep.

The overall aims of analgesia are:

(1) to ensure a satisfactory sleep pattern uninterrupted by pain;

(2) to render the patient pain free while lying in bed or sitting in a chair; and

(3) to provide satisfactory pain relief while the patient is ambulant.

Of these aims, (1) and (2) should be easily obtainable in the majority of patients. (3) is the most difficult and cannot always be achieved.

With attention to detail, therefore, the great majority of pains in malignant diseases can be controlled satisfactorily with a combination of drug therapy and, where indicated, radiotherapy. This leaves only a small minority of patients for whom the more specialised techniques mentioned in the first chapter of this book need to be considered.

Further Reading

The following bibliography is divided into two parts, the first being books that may be immediately available and the second being journal articles and textbooks.

Books

Auton N (1986) Pain: an exploration. Darton, Longman and Todd, London
Bowsher D (1983) In: Lipton S, Miles J (eds) Persistent pain: modern methods of treatment. Vol. 4. Grune and Stratton, New York
Chaitow L (1983) The acupuncture treatment of pain. Thorsons Publishing, Wellingborough
Chard T, Lilford R (1986) Basic sciences for obstetrics and gynaecology, 2nd edn. Springer, Berlin Heidelberg New York
Goldmeier D, Barton S (1987) Sexually transmitted diseases. Springer, Berlin Heidelberg New York
Hull MGR, Joyce DN, Turner G (1986) Undergraduate obstetrics and gynaecology. Wright, Bristol
Jenkins D (1986) Listening to gynaecological patients' problems. Springer, Berlin Heidelberg New York
Ledward RS (1986) Handbook of obstetrics and gynaecology: a guide for housemen. Wright, Bristol
Melzack R, Wall PD (1988) The challenge of pain. Penguin, Harmondsworth
Nicholls J, Glass R (1985) Coloproctology. Springer, Berlin Heidelberg New York
O'Connor DT (1986) Endometriosis. Churchill Livingstone, Edinburgh
Sturdy DE (1986) Outline of urology. Wright, Bristol
Swerdlow M (1986) Therapy of pain, 2nd edn. MTP Press, Lancaster
Willocks J (1978) Essential obstetrics and gynaecology. Churchill Livingstone, Edinburgh
Paulley JW, Pelser HE (1989) Psychological management for psychosomatic disorders. Springer, Berlin Heidelberg New York

Journal Articles and Textbooks

Beard RW, Reginald PW, Pearce S (1986) Pelvic pain in women. Br Med J 293: 1160–1162
Cuschieri A, Giles GR, Moosa AR (eds) (1982) Essential surgical practice. Wright, Bristol
Darougar S (ed) (1983) Chlamydial disease. Br Med Bull 39: 138–150
Decos J, Todd IP (eds) (1988) Anorectal surgery. Churchill Livingstone, Edinburgh
Duguid HLD, Parratt D, Trayhor R (1980) Actinomyces like organisms in cervical smears from women using intrauterine contraceptive devices. Br Med J 281: 534–537
Farquar CM, Beard RW (1988) Pelvic pain. Br J Sexual Med 15: 391–394
Farquar CM, Beard RW (1989) Pelvic pain. Br J Sexual Med 16: 117–123

Fox H (ed) (1987) Haines and Taylor obstetrical and gynaecological pathology, 3rd edn. Churchill Livingstone, Edinburgh

Hibbard BH (ed) (1987) Principles of obstetrics. Butterworth, London

Hughes TJ (1988) A pharmacological basis for the rational use of potent analgesics. Hosp Update 14, 2159–2169

Kass EH (1957) Bacteriuria and the diagnosis of infections of the urinary tract, Arch Intern Med 100: 709–713

Kurman RJ (1989) Blaustein's pathology of the female genital tract, 3rd edn. Springer, Berlin Heidelberg New York

Macfarlane DA, Thomas LP (1984) Textbook of surgery. Churchill Livingstone, Edinburgh

Mardl P, Lind I, Svensson L, Westrom L, Moller BR (1981) Antibodies to *Chlamydia trachomatis*, *Mycoplasma hominis* and *Neisseria gonorrhoeae* in serum from patients with acute salpingitis. Br J Vener Dis 57: 125–129

Maskell R (1988) Urinary tract infection in clinical and laboratory practice, Ch. 4, Edward Arnold, London

Melzack R, Wall PD (1965) Pain mechanism: a new theory. Science 150: 971

Reginald PW, Pearce S, Beard RW (1989) Pelvic pain due to venous congestion. In: Studd J (ed) Progress in obstetrics and gynaecology, vol 7. Churchill Livingstone, Edinburgh

Renaer M (1981) Chronic pelvic pain in women. Springer, Berlin Heidelberg New York

Sparkes RA, Purrier BGA, Watt PJ (1981) Bacteriological colonisation of uterine cavity: role of tailed intra-uterine contraceptive device. Br Med J 282: 1189–1191

Taylor E, Blackwell AL, Barlow D, Phillips J (1982) *Gardnerella vaginalis*: anaerobes and vaginal discharge. Lancet i: 1376–1379

Thomson AD, Cotton RE (1983) Lecture notes on pathology, 3rd edn. Blackwell Scientific, Oxford (1988)

Tindall VR (ed) (1988) Jeffcoate's principles of obstetrics and gynaecology. Butterworth, London

Toth A, O'Leary WM, Ledger W (1982) Evidence for microbial transfer by spermatozoa. Obstet Gynaecol 59: 556–559

Subject Index

Abdomen, acute abdominal crisis 50
Abdomino-pelvic swellings 117–20
Abortion
  missed 73
  pelvic infection following 40'
Abscess
  Bartholin's 83
  Diverticulitis 137
  paracolic 52
  pelvic 126, 134–5
  perianal 87–8
  presacral 52
  psoas 154
  Right iliac fossa 52
  superficial 152
Acquired immune deficiency syndrome
    (AIDS) 35
Actinomycosis 40, 52
Acyclovir 38
Adductor region of pelvis/thigh 154
Adnexa, diagnostic imaging 43
Afferent fibres 7
Age related lower abdominal/pelvic pain
    22
Amenorrhoea 70
Aminoglycoside 40
Amoebic colitis 51
Ampicillin 35
Anaerobes 38, 39
Anal canal
  carcinoma 90–1
  innervation 4
Analgesics 9
Ankylosing spondylitis 55
Anterolateral cordotomy 12
Antidepressants 18, 19
Antiprostaglandins 65, 123
Anxiety
  in gynaecalgia 128–9
  of referral 17
Anxiolytics 18–19

Aortoiliac embolism 148–9
Appendicitis
  acute 133
  chronic 136–7
Arrhenoblastomas 120
Aspirin 65, 157–8

Baclofen 161
Barium enema
  Crohn's disease 51
  colonic spasm 53
  double-contrast 51
  fistulae 52
  large bowel disease 51
  perforation 51
  small bowel 50, 58
Barthinolitis, acute 35
Bartholin's abscess 83
Bartholin's cyst 83
Basal-cell carcinoma 90
Benzhexol 20
Benzodiazepines 18–19
Beta-lactam antibiotic 40
Bilateral oophorectomy 116
Bilateral salpingo-oophorectomy 108
Bladder
  acute pain 93, 94
  calculi 95–6
  carcinoma 98
  chronic pain 93–8
  dysfunction 49
  innervation 3
  pain sensation and discomfort in 93
  schistosomiasis of 95
  tuberculosis 95
  tumours 48
  unstable 97
  see also Cystitis
Bone disorders, metabolic 155
Bone infection 55

Bone pain 161
Bone scintigraphy 55
Bone tumours 55, 155
Buprenorphine 159, 160
Buscopan 143
Buserelin 123

Caecal carcinoma 146–7
Calculi
  bladder 95–6
  pelvic urinary 47–8
  vesical 47–8
Calymmatobacterium granulomatis 37
Cancer
  physical approaches 18
  psychological approach 17–18
Cancerophobia 18, 129
Candida albicans 34, 35
Carbamazepine 19
Carcinoid tumour 50, 52
Cefotaxime 35
Cervical cancer 85
Cervical discharge 40
Cervical erosion 129, 130
Cervical intraepithelial neoplasia 86
Cervicitis 130
  chronic 129
Cervix
  childhood carcinoma of 63
  eversion of 85
Chancroid 37
Chlamydia psittaci 36
Chlamydia trachomatis 36–38, 40
Chlamydial infection 36
Chlorpromazine 20, 161
Chorioncarcinoma 119
Clomipramine 19
Coccydynia 151–2
Coccygeal pain 55
Coccygectomy 152
Codeine 158
Coliforms 38, 39, 61
Colitis 51
Colloid carcinoma 51
Colonic anastomosis 52
Colonic neoplasms 51
Colonic spasm, barium enema 53
Colonoscopy, 26, 146
Colorectal disease 51–2
Colovaginal fistulae 137
Colovesical fistulae 137
Combined oral contraceptive 66, 130
Computed tomography (CT) 48, 52, 54–60
Congenital anomalies of the urinary tract
  49
Congenital malformations, urogenital/
  uterine 62

Constipation, chronic 127, 161
Co-proxamol 158
Corticosteroids 161
Cotrimoxazole 111
Crohn's colitis 51
Crohn's disease 50, 51, 52, 89, 133, 138–9, 141
Cystitis
  chronic 95
  intravenous urography 47
Cystoscopy 25
Cystourethritis, acute 94
Cysts
  Bartholin's 83
  foetal ovarian 62
  ovarian 78, 118–19
  parovarian 78
  vaginal 63
  vulval 63

Danazol 115, 123, 130, 131
Degenerative disease, bone 54
Depression 15, 18, 160
Dermoid, diagnostic tooth of 43
Descending inhibitory augmentation 11–12
Dexamethasone 161
Dextran 58
Dextromoramid 162
Dextropropoxyphene 158
Diagnostic imaging 40–56
  gynaecological disease 41–5
  intestinal disease 49–53
  skeletal disease 54–5
  urinary tract disease 45–9
Diamorphine 161, 160
Diazepam 19, 161
Diethylstilboestrol 85
Dieting 130
Dihydrocodeine 158
Discogenic disease 54
Diverticular disease 137
Diverticulitis 133
Doctor/patient relationship 16, 17
Double-contrast barium enema (DCBE) 51
Double uterus 70
Doxycycline 36
Dyhydrogesterone 67
Dysmenorrhoea 16, 63–8, 121
  causes of 63
  hormonal preparations in 65
  management 65–8
  prostaglandin levels in 64
Dyspareunia 16–17, 40, 68–9, 105, 106,
  110, 128

Ectocervix 85
Ectopic gestation 75–6

Ectopic pregnancy, sonography 45
Electroconvulsive therapy 18
Endometrial carcinoma 85
Endometriosis 112–16, 125
  in pregnancy 78–79
  classification 114
  concept of endometrial bleeding from
    ectopic sites 115
  diagnostic procedures 114–15
  drug effects 116
  medical treatment 115
  pathology of 113
  secondary 116
  sites of 113
  surgical treatment 116
  symptoms 113
Endovaginal scanning 41
Enkephalins 9–10
Enteroureteric fistula 48
Enterovesical fistula 48
Epidural opiates 13
Erythromycin 36, 111
Escherichia coli 31, 47, 83
Ethinyloestradiol 66
Examination
  clinical 24
  general and surgical 21–6
  gynaecological 28–30
  inpatient 25–6
  orthopaedic 30–1
  pelvic 28–30
  rectal 24–5
  vaginal 29

Fallopian tubes, innervation 3–4
Fascia of Denonvilliers 3
Female pelvis. See Pelvis
Femoral neuralgia 154
Fibroma, ovarian 122
Fibromyomata 77–8, 120–2
Fissure in ano
  acute 86–7
  chronic 89
Fistula in ano 89
Flupenthixol decanoate 20
Fluphenazine decanoate 20
Focal bone pain 55

Gardnerella vaginalis 34–5, 83
Genital herpes 35, 37–8
Genital tract tumours 117–20
Genitourinary infections 31–40
Glycine, 58
Gonococcal infection 35
Granuloma inguinale 37
Granulomatous disease 50

Granulosa cell tumours 119
Gut ischaemia 50
Gynaecalgia 127–31
  characteristics of, and features
    associated with 128
  diagnostic investigations 129
  factors influencing experience of 128
Gynaecological disease
  diagnostic imaging 41–5
  preadolescence 59–63
Gynaecological examination 28–30
Gynaecological history 26–8
Gynaecological pain 103–31
Gynaecological problems in pregnancy 77–9

Haemophilus ducreyi 37
Haemorrhoidectomy 87
Haloperidol 161
Hepatitis B 38
Herniae 136
Herpes simplex virus (HSV) 35–7
Hip joint 152–3
History taking 26–7
Hormonal preparations in dysmenorrhoea 65
Hormone replacement therapy 119, 123
Human immunodeficiency viruses 38
Hydronephrosis 126
Hyperparathyroidism 48
Hypnotics 19
Hypogastric plexus 3
Hypogastrium, palpable tumours 148
Hysterectomy 108, 123, 130
  anatomical relations of pelvic viscera
    after 124
  pain after 123–8
  parametrial swelling after 127
Hysteroscopy 58

Ileocaecal disease 52
Iliac vein thrombosis 150
Imidazole 34
Imipramine hydrochloride 97
Infertility 79
Innervation of pelvic viscera 3–5
Intestinal disease, diagnostic imaging 49–53
Intestinal disorders, spasmodic 143
Intestinal fistula, barium examination 52
Intestinal inflammation
  acute 133–4
  chronic 136–62. See also Pelvic
    inflammatory disease
Intestinal ischaemia 135–6
Intestinal obstruction 135–6
Intestinal tract, complicated disease of 52
Intrauterine contraceptive device (IUCD)
  38–9

Intravenous pyelography urography (IVU) 45–7, 62, 126
  preoperative 49
  ureteric disease 48
Investigation, bacteriological 31–40
Irritable bowel syndrome 52–3, 143
Ischaemic colitis 51
Ischial epiphysis, avulsion of 152
Ischiorectal abscess 88

Joint infection 55

Kraurosis vulvae 85

Labour, premature 71–2
Laparoscopy 39, 56–7, 110, 116, 129, 131, 134
Laparotomy 122, 131
Large bowel carcinomas 145–7
Large bowel disease, barium enema 51
Large bowel neoplasms 143–8
Large bowel obstruction 51
Large bowel polyps 51
Left iliac fossa, palpable tumours 148
Leucine enkephalin 10
Leukoplakia 84
Levorphanol 162
Lichen sclerosis 84
Lithium carbonate 19
Local anaesthetic blocks 12
Low back pain 54
Lumbosacral spine 151
Luteinising hormone releasing hormone (LHRH) agonist 115
Lymphogranuloma venereum 36, 37
Lymphosarcoma 50

Malabsorption conditions 50
Meckel's diverticultitis 133
Meckel's diverticulum 50
Medroxyprogesterone 67
Melanoma 90
Menstrual abnormalities 121
Menstruation, family history of 27
Meptazinol 161
Mesodermal sinus tumours 119
Metabolic disorders of bone 155
Metastatic tumours 147
Methionine enkephalin 10
Metronidazole 34, 35, 39, 40, 111
Micturition
  flushing action of 33
  frequency of 70, 94, 110
  frequent and painful 31

Miscarriage
  cause of 74
  diagnosis and management 72
  early 73
  incomplete 73
  presenting signs 74
Monoamine oxidase inhibitors (MAOIs) 19
Morphine 9, 159, 161, 160
Muscle spasms 161
Mycoplasma hominis 36–40
Mycoplasma infections 36–7
Mycoplasma pneumoniae 36
Myeloma 55
Myomectomy 122, 123

Nalbuphine 161
Naloxone 159
Neisseria gonorrhoeae 35, 38–40
Neuralgia paraesthetica 154
Neuromodulation mechanisms 10
Neuropeptides 9–10
Neurosis 15, 19
Nifedipine 67
Night sedation 19
Nitrazepam 19
Nitrofurantoin 33
Nociceptive receptors 6–7
Nocioceptive pathways, interruption of 12
Non-specific vaginitis 34–5
Non-steroidal anti-inflammatory drugs (NSAIDs) 157–8, 161
Norethisterone 66, 67
Nystatin vaginal pessaries 34

Obesity 130
Obsessional disorders 15
Oophorectomy 119, 123, 125
Opiate receptors 9
Opiates 159–61
Orthopaedic examination 30–1
Osteomalacia 155
Osteomyelitis 155
Osteoporosis 55
Ovarian cysts 62, 78, 118–19
Ovarian fibroma 122
Ovarian malignancy 123, 126
Ovarian masses, sonography 43
Ovarian tumours 62–3
Ovary
  in pregnancy 72–3
  innervation 3–4
Oxycodone 162

Paget's disease 55, 155
Pain
  acute 14, 157, 159

anatomophysiology of 6
chronic 14, 157, 160
  benign 160–1
  of malignancy 161–2
conversion 14
expression of 14
intractable 157
management 157–62
mild 157–8
moderate 158
neuroanatomy 6–9
neurogenic 63
neurophysiology of 6–13
physiology 6–9
psychogenic 15
psychology of 14
severe 159–62
sexually related 27
somatic 5, 12
tension 14
threshold of 14
visceral 5, 8–9, 13
see also Pelvic pain
Pain relief 10, 12
Palpable tumours, differential diagnosis of
  147
Papaveretum 160
Paracetamol 65, 157–8
Parametritis 85
Parovarian cysts 78
Pelvic abscess 126, 134–5
Pelvic congestion syndrome 56, 131
Pelvic examination 28–30
Pelvic infection, chronic 40
Pelvic inflammatory disease 38–40, 109–12,
  129
acute 109
antibiotic treatment 111
chronic 110
chronicity of 112
common causes of 111
diagnosis 109
infective agents in 111
management 110, 112
recurrent 110, 111
sonography 44–5
summary of common diagnostic
  specimens 40
Pelvic pain
acute 22
anterior 152–4
chronic 15, 21, 40
  evaluation of symptoms 23–4
  examination for 23–6
  without obvious pathology 17
difficulties in assessment 14–17
gynaecological/obstetric aspects 6

orthopaedic causes of 150–6
posterior 151
psychological aspects of 13–20
surgical aspects 5
surgical causes 133–50
therapeutic implications 16
see also Pain
Pelvic peritoneum, innervation 5
Pelvic swellings 117–20
Pelvic ureter, innervation 5
Pelvic urinary calculi 47–8
Pelvic viscera, innervation 3–5
Pelvirectal tumours, recurrence of 91
Pelvis, anatomy 1–3
Penicillin 35
Pentazocine 159, 160
Perianal abscess 87–8
Perianal haematoma 86
Perineum 86–91
  acute painful conditions 21–2, 86–8
  chronic painful conditions 89–91
Peripheral receptors 6–7
Phenazocine 162
Pilonidal abscess 152
Placental abruption 76–7
Post-hysterectomy syndrome
  management 125
  pain 123
Polycystic ovary syndrome 49
Polypoidal masses 51
Prednisone 141
Pregnancy 69–79
  abnormalities of 73–4
  ectopic 75–6
  failures of 73
  fear of 69
  gynaecological problems in 77–9
  ovary in 72–3
  pelvic examination 71
  physiological discomforts of 71
  tests 74
  trophoblastic disease in 74–5
  uterine contractility in 71–2
  uterine enlargement in 120–3
Premenstrual tension 16, 129
Presacral abscess 52
Presacral neurectomy 67
Probenecid 35
Procaine penicillin 35
Prochlorperazine 161
Procidentia 103–4
Proctalgia fugax 143
Proctoscopy 25
Progesterone 67
Progestogens 66–7, 115, 123, 130, 131
Prolapsed internal pile 87
Propantheline bromide 97

Prostaglandin levels in dysmenorrhoea 64
Proximal hamstring injury 152
Proximal thigh 154
Psoas abscess 154
Psychiatric illness 15, 16
Psychoactive drugs 16
Psychological support 130, 131
Psychosexual problems 126
Psychosomatic medicine 13–14
Psychotropic drugs 20
Pyelonephritis, acute 33

Radiation colitis 51
Radiation ileitis 50
Radiological intervention techniques 56
Rape 69, 81
Rectal carcinoma 52
Rectal examination 24–5
Rectal inflammation 51
Rectal prolapse 89–90
  adult 90
  infantile 90
Rectosigmoidoscopy 25
Rectum
  adenomas of 143–5
  innervation 4
Rectus abdominis insertion injury 153
Rectus femoris insertion injury 154
Recurrent tumours 147
Relaxation 19
Reproduction 59–79
Right iliac fossa, palpable tumours 148

Sacrococcygeal pain 151–2
Sacroiliac joint
  pain in 151
  septic arthritis of 155
Sacroiliitis 55
Salpingitis 133
  acute 35, 36, 38–40
Schistosoma haematobium 95
Schistosomiasis 47
Schizophrenia 15, 18, 20
Segmental modulation augmentation 10–11
Sexual abuse 59
Sexual activity 61, 68–79, 126, 129
Sexual assault 82
Sexual experience 126
Sexual fantasy 130
Sexual intercourse 31, 34
Sexually related pain 27
Sexually transmitted disease 35–8, 82, 83
Sigmoid colon
  adenomas of 143–5
  carcinoma 146

Sigmoidoscopy 51, 139
Skeletal disease, diagnostic imaging
  54–5
Small bowel disease
  adenocarcinoma 50
  adhesions 50
  barium enema 50, 58
  herniation 50
  primary tumours 50
Small bowel obstruction 50
Sodium valproate 160, 161
Somatic pain 5, 12
Sonography
  ectopic pregnancy 45
  gynaecological disease 41
  ovarian masses 43
  pelvic inflammatory disease 44–5
  uterus 42–3
Spectinomycin 35
Sphincter spasms 161
Spina bifida 54
Spina bifida occulta 54
Spinal cord
  ascending pathways 8
  descending inhibitory mechanism 7
  segmental mechanism 7
Spondylolysthesis 54
Squamous cell carcinomas 90
Staphylococcal infection 61
Staphylococcus saprophyticus 31
Stoma management 142–3
Streptococcus pyogenes 35
Stress effects 130
Substance P 10
Sulphasalazine 141
Sympathetic block 13
Symphysis pubis 153
Syphilis 37

Temazepam 19
Terramycin 111
Testosterone 67
Tetracycline 36, 39
Thrombosed external pile 86
Thrombosis 148–9
Toxic megacolon 51
Tranquillisers 20
Tranylcypromine 19
Trauma in preadolescence 61
Trichomonas vaginalis 34–5, 83
Trifluoperazine 20
Trigonitis 85
Trimethoprim 33
Trophoblastic disease in pregnancy 74–5
Tuberculosis 40, 47, 50, 52, 95
Tuberculous colitis 51

Ulcerative colitis 89, 140–1
Ulcerative proctocolitis, 139–42
  carcinoma 140
Ultrasonography 42, 49, 52, 62, 77, 119,
  131
Ureaplasma urealyticans 36–7
Ureteric colic 99–100
Ureteric disease, intravenous urography 48
Ureteic displacement 126–7
Ureteric obstruction 93, 99
Ureteric pain 93, 99–101
  acute 99–100
  chronic 99, 101
Ureterocele 47
Urethra, innervation 3
Urethral caruncle 93–4
Urethral syndrome 31
Urinalysis 25
Urinary fistula to the vagina 48
Urinary tract, congenital anomalies 49
Urinary tract disease, diagnostic imaging
  45–9
Urinary tract infection 31–4, 134
  intravenous urography 47
  postoperative 125
Urine culture 33
Urine retention
  acute 94
  chronic 94–5
  pregnancy 70
Uterine contractility in pregnancy 71–2
Uterine enlargement
  causes of 122
  in pregnancy 120–3
  management 123
Uterine fibroids/fibromyomata 77, 121, 122
Uterovaginal prolapse 103–5
Uterus
  anteflexed retroposition 106
  congenital anomalies 62
  double 70
  innervation 3–4

malposition 105–9
normal position of anteflexion and
  anteversion 105
retroflexed retroversion 70, 105, 106
retroversion 69, 114, 129, 130
sonography 42–3

Vagina
  adenosis 85
  infections 82–4
  innervation 3–4
  shortening of 126
  trauma 81–2
Vaginal cervix 85–6
Vaginal cysts 63
Vaginal discharge 34–5, 59, 63, 81, 109,
  110, 125
Vaginal dryness 127
Vaginal examination 29
Vaginal infections 59–61
Vaginal transducers 41
Vaginal tumours 85
Vaginal vault granulation tissue 126
Vaginismus 17
Vaginitis, non-specific 34–5
Vascular disorders 148–9
Venography 150
Vesical calculi 47–8
Vesical tumour 48
Vesicorectal adhesion 126
Villous ademoma 144
Vulva
  infections 82–4
  trauma 81–2
Vulval carcinoma-in-situ 84
Vulval cysts 63
Vulval dystrophy/dermatoses 84–5
Vulval haematoma 82
Vulval infections 59–61
Vulval tumours 84
Vulvovaginal laceration 61